Curbside Consultation
in Pediatric Neurology

49 Clinical Questions

Curbside Consultation in Pediatrics
SERIES

SERIES EDITOR, LISA B. ZAOUTIS, MD

Curbside Consultation
in Pediatric Neurology

49 Clinical Questions

EDITORS

Daniel J. Licht, MD
Associate Professor of Neurology and Pediatrics
The Children's Hospital of Philadelphia
Perelman School of Medicine
University of Pennsylvania
Philadelphia, Pennsylvania

Nicole R. Ryan, MD
Division of Neurology
The Children's Hospital of Philadelphia
Philadelphia, Pennsylvania

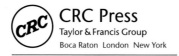 **CRC Press**
Taylor & Francis Group
Boca Raton London New York

CRC Press is an imprint of the
Taylor & Francis Group, an **informa** business

First published 2016 by SLACK Incorporated

Published 2024 by CRC Press
2385 NW Executive Center Drive, Suite 320, Boca Raton FL 33431

and by CRC Press
4 Park Square, Milton Park, Abingdon, Oxon, OX14 4RN

CRC Press is an imprint of Taylor & Francis Group, LLC

© 2016 Taylor & Francis Group, LLC

Library of Congress Cataloging-in-Publication Data

Curbside consultation in pediatric neurology : 49 clinical questions / Daniel Licht, Nicole R. Ryan.
    p. ; cm. -- (Curbside consultation in pediatrics)
  Includes bibliographical references and index.
  ISBN 978-1-61711-599-8 (paperback)
  I. Licht, Daniel J., author, editor. II. Ryan, Nicole R., author, editor. III. Title. IV. Series: Curbside consultation in pediatrics series
  [DNLM: 1. Nervous System Diseases--diagnosis. 2. Nervous System Diseases--therapy. 3. Child. 4. Pediatrics--methods. WS 340]
  RJ506.N48
  618.92'80076--dc23
                        2015012936

ISBN: 9781617115998 (pbk)
ISBN: 9781003523659 (ebk)

DOI: 10.1201/9781003523659

Dedication

To Midori, Stefano, and Massimo—
thank you for all your support and love.

—DJL

To Sean and Zoe—
Your love and support keep me going. Thank you!

—NRR

Contents

About the Editors

Daniel J. Licht, MD is a child neurologist with expertise in critical care neurology, stroke, and noninvasive imaging. Dr. Licht started his career as a synthetic organic chemist after completing his bachelor's degree in biochemistry at NYU in 1984. He graduated from New Jersey Medical School (UMDNJ) in 1997 and began his second (and final) career as a pediatric resident at The Children's Hospital of Philadelphia, following into a neurology residency at the University of Pennsylvania.

Nicole R. Ryan, MD is a child neurologist and epileptologist at The Children's Hospital of Philadelphia. After completing a bachelor's degree in psychology at Cornell University, she entered the Albert Einstein School of Medicine where she discovered her passion for neurology. She completed her residency training at the Perelman School of Medicine and has stayed on at The Children's Hospital of Philadelphia as the Section Head of Community Neurology and member of the Pediatric Regional Epilepsy Program.

Contributing Authors

Laura A. Adang, MD, PhD (Questions 17, 43)
Division of Child Neurology
The Children's Hospital of Philadelphia
Philadelphia, Pennsylvania

Robert A. Avery, DO, MSCE (Questions 37, 38)
Center for Neuroscience and Behavior
Children's National Medical Center
Washington, DC

Ernest Barbosa, MD (Question 12)
The Children's Hospital of Philadelphia
Philadelphia, Pennsylvania

David Bearden, MD (Question 41)
Division of Child Neurology
The Children's Hospital of Philadelphia
Philadelphia, Pennsylvania

Timothy J. Bernard, MD, MSCS (Question 36)
Director, Pediatric Stroke Program
Associate Professor of Pediatrics,
    Neurology and Child Neurology
University of Colorado School of Medicine
Director of Clinical Research, Children's
    Clinical Research Organization
Children's Hospital Colorado
    Research Institute
Associate Director, Pediatric Neurology
    Residency Program
Children's Hospital Colorado
Aurora, Colorado

Lauren A. Beslow, MD, MSCE (Question 34)
Assistant Professor of
    Pediatrics and Neurology
Director
Pediatric and Neonatal Stroke Program
Yale University School of Medicine
New Haven, Connecticut

Diana X. Bharucha-Goebel, MD (Question 31)
Children's National Medical Center
Washington, DC

Lori L. Billinghurst, MD, MSc, FRCPC
    (Question 34)
Clinical Assistant Professor of Neurology
Perelman School of Medicine
University of Pennsylvania
Attending Physician
The Children's Hospital of Philadelphia
Philadelphia, Pennsylvania

John M. Binder, MD (Question 36)
Pediatric Neurology
Children's Hospital Colorado
Aurora, Colorado
Billings Clinic
Billings, Montana

Jason Coryell, MD, MS (Question 6)
Oregon Health & Sciences University
Portland, Oregon

Louis T. Dang, MD, PhD (Question 33)
Division of Pediatric Neurology
Department of Pediatrics
University of Michigan
Ann Arbor, Michigan

Mai T. Dang, MD, PhD (Questions 12, 45)
Division of Neurology
The Children's Hospital of Philadelphia
Philadelphia, Pennsylvania

Emily A. Gertsch, MD, MPH (Question 8)
Department of Neurology
Boston Children's Hospital
Boston, Massachusetts

Ethan M. Goldberg, MD, PhD (Question 44)
Attending Physician
Division of Neurology
The Children's Hospital of Philadelphia
Philadelphia, Pennsylvania

Matthew Grady, MD, FAAP, CAQSM
    (Question 29)
Fellowship Director
Primary Care Sports Medicine
Assistant Professor of Clinical Pediatrics
Perelman School of Medicine
University of Pennsylvania
Pediatric and Adolescent Sports Medicine
Department of Orthopedic Surgery
The Children's Hospital of Philadelphia
Philadelphia, Pennsylvania

Adam L. Hartman, MD (Question 7)
Associate Professor of
    Neurology and Pediatrics
Johns Hopkins University
Attending Physician
Johns Hopkins Hospital
Baltimore, Maryland

Daphne M. Hasbani, MD, PhD (Question 2)
Section of Child Neurology
St. Christopher's Hospital for Children
Assistant Clinical Professor
Drexel University College of Medicine
Philadelphia, Pennsylvania

Amanda L. Hollatz, MA (Question 36)
Pediatrics
Hemophilia & Thrombosis Center
University of Colorado School of Medicine
Aurora, Colorado

Matthew P. Kirschen, MD, PhD
    (Questions 28, 30)
Departments of Anesthesia and
    Critical Care Medicine and Neurology
The Children's Hospital of Philadelphia
Philadelphia, Pennsylvania

Kelly Knupp, MD (Question 8)
Assistant Professor of
    Pediatrics and Neurology
University of Colorado—
    Anschutz Medical Campus
Division of Pediatric Neurology
Children's Hospital Colorado
Aurora, Colorado

Steven Kugler, MD (Question 18)
Attending Neurologist
The Children's Hospital of Philadelphia
Chalfont, Pennsylvania

Ronald F. Marchese, MD (Question 28)
Assistant Professor
Department of Pediatrics
Perelman School of Medicine
University of Pennsylvania
Division of Emergency Medicine
The Children's Hospital of Philadelphia
Philadelphia, Pennsylvania

Brian Masselink, MD (Question 7)
Resident
Pediatric Neurology
Johns Hopkins Hospital
Baltimore, Maryland

Christina L. Master, MD, FAAP, CAQSM
    (Question 27)
Associate Professor of Clinical Pediatrics
Perelman School of Medicine
University of Pennsylvania
Pediatric and Adolescent Sports Medicine
Division of Pediatric Orthopedics
Associate Program Director
Primary Care Sports Medicine Fellowship
Attending Physician
Care Network—Karabots Center
The Children's Hospital of Philadelphia
Philadelphia, Pennsylvania

Jennifer L. McGuire, MD, MSCE
    (Questions 26, 32)
Instructor of Neurology
Division of Neurology
The Children's Hospital of Philadelphia
Department of Neurology
Perelman School of Medicine
University of Pennsylvania
Philadelphia, Pennsylvania

Kashif Ali Mir, MD (Question 11)
Child Neurology Fellow
Division of Pediatric Neurology
Department of Neurology
University of Louisville School of Medicine
Louisville, Kentucky

John R. Mytinger, MD (Question 5)
Assistant Professor
The Ohio State University
Director
Infantile Spasms Program
Nationwide Children's Hospital
Columbus, Ohio

*Xilma R. Ortiz-Gonzalez, MD, PhD
    (Questions 15, 46)*
Division of Neurology
Department of Pediatrics
The Children's Hospital of Philadelphia
Philadelphia, Pennsylvania

Jessica A. Panzer, MD, PhD (Question 48)
Division of Neurology
Department of Pediatrics
The Children's Hospital of Philadelphia
Department of Neurology
Perelman School of Medicine
University of Pennsylvania
Philadelphia, Pennsylvania

Alyssa Pensirikul, MD (Question 39)
Assistant Professor of Clinical Neurology
University of Miami
Miami, Florida

Emily Robbins, MD (Question 19)
The Children's Hospital of Philadelphia
Philadelphia, Pennsylvania

Caitlin Rollins, MD (Question 14)
Department of Neurology
Boston Children's Hospital
Boston, Massachusetts

Alyssa R. Rosen, MD (Question 40)
Division of Pediatric Neurology
Department of Pediatrics
The Children's Hospital of Philadelphia
Philadelphia, Pennsylvania

Joyce Sapin, MD (Question 20)
Attending Neurologist
The Children's Hospital of Philadelphia
Philadelphia, Pennsylvania

Renée A. Shellhaas, MD, MS (Question 33)
Clinical Associate Professor
Division of Pediatric Neurology
Department of Pediatrics
University of Michigan
Ann Arbor, Michigan

*Maximillian H. Shmidheiser, PsyD, ABPP-CN
    (Question 30)*
Clinical Neuropsychologist
MossRehab Concussion Center and
    Drucker Brain Injury Center
MossRehab Hospital
Wynnewood, Pennsylvania

Laufey Yr Sigurdardottir, MD (Questions 9, 47)
Director of Epilepsy Services
Nemours Children's Hospital
Orlando, Florida

Karen L. Skjei, MD (Questions 10, 11)
Assistant Professor
Division of Pediatric Neurology
Department of Neurology
University of Louisville School of Medicine
Louisville, Kentucky

Douglas Smith, MD (Question 16)
Division of Neurology
The Children's Hospital of Philadelphia
Philadelphia, Pennsylvania

Donna J. Stephenson, MD (Questions 13, 49)
Assistant Professor of Neurology
The Children's Hospital of Philadelphia
Philadelphia, Pennsylvania

Christina Szperka, MD (Questions 16, 19)
Director
Pediatric Headache Program
The Children's Hospital of Philadelphia
Philadelphia, Pennsylvania

Katherine S. Taub, MD (Question 4)
Assistant Professor
Perelman School of Medicine
University of Pennsylvania
Pediatric Epileptologist
The Children's Hospital of Philadelphia
Philadelphia, Pennsylvania

J. Michael Taylor, MD (Question 38)
Assistant Professor of Neurology
Cincinnati Children's Hospital
    Medical Center
Cincinnati, Ohio

*Christian Turner, MD, FAAP, CAQSM
    (Question 29)*
Department of Orthopedic Surgery
The Children's Hospital of Philadelphia
Philadelphia, Pennsylvania

Amy T. Waldman, MD, MSCE (Question 42)
Assistant Professor of Neurology
The Children's Hospital of Philadelphia
Philadelphia, Pennsylvania

Ryan P. Williams, MD, EdM (Question 3)
Division of Neurology
The Children's Hospital of Philadelphia
Philadelphia, Pennsylvania

Courtney J. Wusthoff, MD, MS (Question 35)
Division of Child Neurology
Stanford University
Palo Alto, California

Michele L. Yang, MD (Questions 24, 25)
Assistant Professor
Department of Pediatrics and Neurology
Children's Hospital Colorado
Aurora, Colorado

Sabrina W. Yum, MD (Question 23)
Division of Neurology
The Children's Hospital of Philadelphia
Department of Neurology
Perelman School of Medicine
University of Pennsylvania
Philadelphia, Pennsylvania

Introduction

The neurological exam of children is challenging, as children may not be able to follow commands or answer questions to help inform the clinician. Trickery, observation, and a deep understanding of the expected responses are the skills needed. This text has been prepared to help pediatricians, medical students, parents, and other non-neurologists understand the presentation and basic care for the most common neurological problems. Each question (chapter) is designed to take the reader from the complaint symptoms for each problem, to developing a differential diagnosis, and then treatment considerations. Each question was analyzed and reported on with up-to-date information and expert insight. Furthermore, we hope to impart knowledge that will lead to the recognition of complaints that need urgent referral from more simple presentations that can be managed by the first-line provider. We took great care to ensure that the text was written in a succinct, but clear and enjoyable manner, with tables that are easy to use and informative.

Daniel J. Licht, MD
Nicole R. Ryan, MD

SECTION I

SEIZURES

HOW ARE SEIZURES CLASSIFIED?

Nicole R. Ryan, MD

The ability to appropriately classify patients with recurrent seizures has far-reaching implications. Our ability to communicate with one another, to discuss prognoses with families, and to choose correct treatment hinges on a universal, clearly stated classification system. As our understanding of genetics and advanced imaging techniques moves forward, the complexity of such a classification system expands. There have been recent attempts to revise older systems to reflect this scientific progress, leading to controversy as old concepts and familiar terms are abandoned. When thinking about a particular patient with epilepsy, it has been proposed to describe him or her based on clinical features, etiology or epilepsy syndrome, and age of onset (Table 1-1).

Clinical Features

In the past, the terms *partial* and *focal* have referred to seizures that presumably originate from one part of the brain, as compared to generalized seizures, which involve the entire cortex at onset. As having 2 terms referring to the same concept is confusing, focal has replaced partial. There has also been controversy as to the utility of the terms *simple* and *complex*. Simple refers to a seizure in which consciousness is preserved whereas complex refers to a seizure in which consciousness is lost. It has been suggested that focal seizures be described according to their characteristics rather than relying solely on the confusing terms simple or complex. For example, a seizure could be described as "focal with impairment of consciousness" or "focal with subjective sensory symptoms only (ie, aura)." It can also be difficult to determine the state of consciousness of some patients during a seizure.

Licht DJ, Ryan NR, eds. *Curbside Consultation in Pediatric Neurology: 49 Clinical Questions* (pp 3-5).
© 2016 Taylor & Francis Group.

Table 1-1
Clinical Features, Etiology, and Age at Onset of Epilepsy

Clinical Features	Etiology	Age at Onset
Generalized seizures	Genetic	Neonatal (< 44 weeks' gestation)
Tonic-clonic	Structural/metabolic	Infant (< 1 year)
Tonic	Unknown	Child (1 to 12 years)
Clonic		Adolescent (12 to 18 years)
Absence		Adult (> 18 years)
Myoclonic		
Atonic		
Focal seizures		
Unknown		

Generalized seizures can also be further subclassified. The most commonly recognized type of seizure in popular media is a generalized tonic-clonic seizure or "grand mal." Tonic refers to stiffening of the body whereas clonic refers to rhythmic, jerking movements of the extremities. Seizures can also be tonic alone without a clonic component or atonic, which refers to a loss of tone, often leading to a patient falling to the ground. A myoclonic seizure involves a rapid jerking movement of the body. An absence seizure ("petit mal") is probably the most commonly confused type of generalized seizure. It typically involves an arrest of activity with staring lasting several seconds with an immediate return to baseline. Absence seizures can be triggered by hyperventilation and this is performed during an electroencephalogram (EEG) to help make the diagnosis. The seizure is sometimes associated with unusual blinking or nonpurposeful hand movements (automatisms). While focal seizures may also involve some of these features, they are typically longer and have a post-ictal period. Many patients claim to have absence seizures when in reality they have focal seizures, which dramatically alters treatment decisions. It is also important to remember that not all staring is seizures. More commonly, you are dealing with an inattentive child. When in doubt, it is also extremely helpful to obtain a video of a particular event or seizure. In a child with frequent falls, for example, a video may help you determine if the child is falling to the ground because of a sudden body jerk (myoclonic), a loss of tone (atonic), or possibly a nonepileptic cause, such as incoordination.

Etiology of Seizures and Epilepsy Syndromes

It has long been recognized that certain patients with epilepsy share similar characteristics. This has led to the designation of seizure "syndromes." These syndromes are often defined based on age at onset, delayed or normal development, EEG features, provoking factors, or relationship to sleep/wake cycles. For example, patients with childhood absence epilepsy tend to have onset between 4 and 10 years of age, have otherwise normal development, and have a classic 3-hertz generalized spike and wave pattern on EEG that can be induced by hyperventilation. Over time, some of these syndromes have been determined to have a genetic basis (ie, sodium channel, voltage-gated, type I, alpha subunit (*SCN1A*) mutations in patients with Dravet syndrome) while others were defined more by a structural abnormality (ie, mesial temporal lobe epilepsy).

Given the high number of different epilepsy syndromes, it has been proposed that epilepsy be described as either genetic, structural/metabolic, or of unknown cause. In order for an epilepsy to be considered genetic, there must be a known or presumed genetic defect of which seizures are a primary symptom. A structural cause is any visible change on brain imaging that leads to onset of seizures such as trauma, stroke, arteriovenous malformation, or a malformation of cortical development. Epilepsies of unknown cause may be suspected to have a genetic basis but no specific abnormality has been identified. It is likely that several epilepsy syndromes will move between categories as further advances are made.

Age at Onset

Certain electroclinical syndromes are also known to start within certain age groups, and documenting the age of onset may provide further insight into the type of epilepsy and possibly the prognosis for an individual patient. It has been proposed that ages be grouped as neonatal (< 44 weeks' gestational age), infant (< 1 year), child (1 to 12 years), adolescent (12 to 18 years), and adult (> 18 years). As mentioned earlier, childhood absence epilepsy typically begins between 4 and 10 years of age with children often outgrowing seizures by adolescence. Another electroclinical syndrome, juvenile absence epilepsy, involves the same seizure type but starts in adolescence and carries a prognosis of lifelong seizures so age at onset becomes extremely important.

Pulling It All Together

It has probably now become apparent that developing a universal classification system is complicated and needs to be flexible. When conveying information about one of your patients, rather than just referring to a child with "seizures," you should now be able to state that your patient has, for example, "focal epilepsy with impairment of consciousness of unknown cause and childhood onset." Should you classify a child as having "infantile onset epilepsy with myoclonic and generalized tonic-clonic seizures often provoked by fever," you would be giving a very suggestive description of a child with Dravet syndrome. By using common language, we will be better able to communicate with each other and help families start to understand their child's symptoms and ultimate prognosis.

Suggested Readings

Berg AT, Berkovic SF, Brodie MJ, et al. Revised terminology and concepts for organization of seizures and epilepsies: report of the ILAE Commission on Classification and Terminology, 2005-2009. *Epilepsia.* 2010;51:676-685.

Berg AT, Scheffer IE. New concepts in classification of the epilepsies: entering the 21st century. *Epilepsia.* 2011;52:1058-1062.

Panayiotopoulos C. The new ILAE report on terminology and concepts for the organization of epilepsies: critical review and contribution. *Epilepsia.* 2012;53(3):399-404.

How Do I Distinguish Syncope From Seizure?

Daphne M. Hasbani, MD, PhD

Episodic loss of consciousness is a common reason for referral to a pediatric neurology or epilepsy clinic. Differentiating between seizure and syncope is a frequently encountered clinical scenario that impacts subsequent workup and treatment. Because these episodes tend to occur infrequently with each patient, you will most often be making a diagnosis based solely on the history of the event. Therefore, you should take a very detailed step-by-step history of the sequence of events surrounding these episodes.

Precipitating events must be elicited. What was the patient doing just before the event? Did he just stand up? Was she exercising? Was he just using the bathroom (either micturition or defecation) prior to the event? Was it a hot day? Was she having blood drawn? Was there a provoking stressor or significant associated anxiety/crying with hyperventilation? These are all common precipitating factors to syncope. True reflex seizures, or seizures in response to specific precipitating factors, are rare, and the precipitating events are almost never the ones that precede syncope. As a general rule, seizures can occur at any time of day or night, while it is extremely rare for syncope to occur out of sleep.

Prodromal symptoms are common in syncope and are termed *presyncope*. These include feelings of lightheadedness, dizziness, or vertigo. Sufferers of presyncope commonly describe vision changes including graying, going black, tunneling, or becoming blurry. Some patients describe nausea, feeling hot and sweaty, heart racing, or palpitations. Others describe abdominal pain or tingling of the extremities. While all of these symptoms can be associated with seizures in rare situations, they are far more likely to be indicative of syncope. Focal prodromal symptoms such as facial droop or unilateral arm shaking should make you suspicious for seizure or other acute neurologic disorder rather than syncope.

Tongue biting, particularly the sides of the tongue, is commonly reported with seizures but is not a typical feature of syncope. A recent study found that tongue biting had a sensitivity of

Licht DJ, Ryan NR, eds. *Curbside Consultation in Pediatric Neurology: 49 Clinical Questions* (pp 7-9).
© 2016 Taylor & Francis Group.

33% with a specificity of 96% in the diagnosis of seizures.[1] In contrast, urinary incontinence is commonly reported both in seizure and syncope, and another recently published study by the same group found that the presence of urinary incontinence had no value in the differentiation between seizures and syncope.[2]

Patients with syncope will almost always go limp or lose tone as they become unconscious. Bystanders often describe eyes rolling up in the head followed by eye closure during the period of unconsciousness. Occasionally, patients with syncope will stiffen and even convulse, sometimes with focal myoclonic movements.[3] This "convulsive syncope" is more common when patients are kept in a more upright position during the period of unconsciousness. Convulsions following syncope are brief, on the order of a few seconds, whereas they are usually longer with seizures. Eyes are typically open during generalized convulsive seizures. Furthermore, syncopal convulsions are not associated with significant post-event confusion.

The duration of the unconscious period is usually short with syncope, on average less than 30 seconds. In contrast, unconsciousness can be this short during seizures but is often longer, on the order of a few minutes. The duration of loss of consciousness can be prolonged in patients with syncope if they are kept in an upright position.

What happens once the patient regains consciousness? It is normal to feel a little "out of it" after syncope. Most patients with syncope will be confused as to what just happened, but they should be able to articulate this in a clear way. In contrast, the post-ictal confusion that accompanies a seizure is typically more pronounced. In this case, patients are often not able to speak clearly or at all, may be combative, or may remain lethargic and difficult to arouse. Patients with seizures often complain of post-ictal headache, whereas this is infrequent with syncope except in cases where patients are prone to headache such as with migraine sufferers. Profound fatigue requiring a period of sleep is less common after syncope than seizure. Focal complaints such as unilateral arm weakness or facial droop following an event should alert you to something other than syncope. Finally, the duration of post-ictal symptoms should be brief with syncope, on the order of several seconds to minutes, whereas this is typically minutes to hours following a seizure.

I recommend judicious use of diagnostic testing only after you have taken a thorough history. If the event sounds like syncope, orthostatic vital signs can easily be obtained in the office, and presyncopal symptoms can often be provoked with this test. Electrocardiogram should be performed in any patient presenting with suspected syncope to evaluate for potentially dangerous or fatal cardiac arrhythmias. Tilt table testing, Holter monitoring, and implantable loop recorders can also be used to evaluate the etiology of syncope but should not be used to make the initial diagnosis. Electroencephalogram (EEG) should be performed only once the patient is referred to a neurologist who can properly interpret the results in the appropriate clinical context. EEG is only clearly diagnostic for seizure if a typical clinical event is captured during the test, although there are some EEG patterns that may suggest that a patient is prone to seizures. It is important to keep in mind, however, that up to 3.5% of the nonepileptic pediatric population has an interictal EEG abnormality, and many patients with epilepsy have normal interictal EEGs.[4] Thus, caution should be taken not to rely too heavily on the results of diagnostic testing. Brain imaging should be performed only if the history suggests seizure rather than syncope or if the neurologic exam is abnormal. These diagnostic tests are most valuable in the context of a high pretest probability for seizure, and most errors in diagnosis occur when clinicians rely more on diagnostic testing than on the history. The historical features described above should help prevent you from falling into the same trap.

References

1. Brigo F, Nardone R, Ausserer H, et al. The diagnostic value of urinary incontinence in the differential diagnosis of seizures. *Seizure*. 2013;22(2):85-90.
2. Brigo F, Nardone R, Bongiovanni LG. Value of tongue biting in the differential diagnosis between epileptic seizures and syncope. *Seizure*. 2012;21(8):568-572.
3. Lempert T, Bauer M, Schmidt D. Syncope: a videometric analysis of 56 episodes of transient cerebral hypoxia. *Ann Neurol*. 1994;36:233-237.
4. Zivin L, Marsan CA. Incidence and prognostic significance of "epileptiform" activity in the EEG of non-epileptic subjects. *Brain*. 1968;91(4):751-778.

ARE CHILDREN WITH FEBRILE SEIZURES AT GREATER RISK FOR EPILEPSY? WHICH OF THESE PATIENTS SHOULD BE REFERRED TO A NEUROLOGIST?

Ryan P. Williams, MD, EdM

When I see a child in the clinic, emergency room, or pediatric ward with a chief complaint of febrile seizure, I often find the child appearing relatively well but the family in various stages of anxiety. The paroxysmal nature of febrile seizures catches parents unaware. They assumed that their child had acquired a viral or other mild infection with a predictable medical course. Suddenly, however, the child had a seizure. Many questions are whirling around their heads but one of the most anxiety provoking is, "Will my previously well child now have epilepsy?" This is, obviously, a crucial question for parents and one that both the child neurologist and the pediatrician should be well equipped to answer. Unsurprisingly, the answer is complicated and involves variables such as age, family history, and neurodevelopmental status.

In guiding parents of children with only febrile seizures, I find it helpful to immediately reassure them that their child currently does not have epilepsy, which is defined as 2 or more unprovoked (nonfebrile) seizures. Following this reassurance, I ask about the semiology of the seizure, whether it was a first-time febrile seizure, and if there is a family history of febrile seizures and/or epilepsy. Additionally, I delve into the child's developmental history, as children with developmental delays have a higher risk of neurological illness, including epilepsy.

Semiology is key in determining both acute management and prognosis. Febrile seizures are most commonly categorized as one of 2 possible subtypes: simple and complex. Prolonged febrile seizures or febrile status epilepticus (lasting > 30 minutes) is a medical emergency and considered as separate from the usually self-resolving simple and complex febrile seizures.

According to the American Academy of Pediatrics (AAP),[1] a simple febrile seizure is defined as a generalized, nonfocal seizure lasting less than 15 minutes and occurring in the context of a febrile illness in a child between the ages of 6 months and 6 years of age. Most febrile seizures last less than 5 minutes and self-resolve. A complex febrile seizure, in contrast, has focal neurological signs, lasts longer than 15 minutes, and/or occurs more than once in a 24-hour period.

Licht DJ, Ryan NR, eds. *Curbside Consultation in Pediatric Neurology: 49 Clinical Questions* (pp 11-14).
© 2016 Taylor & Francis Group.

Table 3-1

Emergency Management of Simple Febrile Seizures by Age

Age	*Lumbar Puncture*	*Electroencephalogram*	*Imaging*
6 to 12 months	Consider if (1) child is not immunized against *Haemophilus influenzae* type b (Hib) or *Streptococcus pneumoniae,* or (2) clinically warranted	Not recommended	Not recommended
12 months to 6 years	Consider if clinically warranted	Not recommended	Not recommended

---

Focal neurological signs are symptoms such as unilateral extremity stiffening or jerking that can be mapped to a particular location in the brain. Of note, there is a common misperception that eye deviation is a sufficient sign of neurologic focality; in fact, there are both ipsilateral and contralateral gaze centers and, thus, while eye deviation may be an element of focality, it is neither necessary nor sufficient in establishing a neuroanatomical seizure focus.[2]

After determining febrile seizure subtype, I have a baseline from which to start developing a prognosis. Multiple studies[3,4] have shown that most children with simple febrile seizures have an insignificant increased risk of developing epilepsy compared to that of the general population (2.4% vs 1.4%). This appears to be the case regardless of either the number of simple febrile seizures that occur in early childhood or a family history of febrile or afebrile seizures. Care should be taken when interpreting family history data as genetic epilepsies that include febrile seizures (ie, sodium channel, voltage-gated, type I, alpha subunit [*SCN1A*]) had not been discovered at the time of these studies. Therefore, I would expect that there is a stronger relationship between febrile seizures and epilepsy in some families.[3] Thus, you can provide reassurance to parents of children with simple febrile seizures that the risk of future afebrile seizures is low. I do, nonetheless, inform parents that their child may have additional febrile seizures, especially if they are toward the younger age range during their first presentation. In fact, in children less than 12 months who have a simple febrile seizure, the risk of subsequent febrile seizures is 50%. Children who are 12 months or older when they present with a febrile seizure have a slightly lower (30%) recurrence risk; however, that risk increases to 50% after a second febrile seizure. Once again, however, these recurrent febrile seizures do not give the child a diagnosis of epilepsy and neither referral to a child neurologist nor electrodiagnostic (electroencephalogram [EEG]) or imaging evaluation is necessary (see Table 3-1 for suggestions on emergency management of simple febrile seizures).

Nonetheless, despite the known patterns of recurrence, parents and pediatricians alike have understandable concerns when children have multiple episodes of simple febrile seizures. Many clinicians would prefer neurologist input in these cases. I would suggest a child neurology

---

Table 3-2

Emergency Management of Complex Febrile Seizures (Excluding Febrile Status Epilepticus) by Age

Age	Lumbar Puncture	Electroencephalogram	Imaging
6 to 12 months	Recommended	Recommended as outpatient	MRI recommended as outpatient
12 months to 6 years	Consider if clinically warranted	Recommended as outpatient	MRI recommended as outpatient

evaluation of a developmentally normal child (atypically developing children require a different approach) only if the following factors are present: (1) febrile seizure onset at less than 7 months; (2) 5 or greater febrile seizures prior to 1 year of age; and (3) a history of prolonged febrile seizures lasting 10 minutes or longer. Children with these factors are more likely (positive predictive value [PPV] of 88% to 94%) to have a specific genetic mutation causing a sodium channelopathy (*SCN1A*) that accounts for their febrile seizures and dramatically increases their risk of epilepsy.[5-7] I will address the associations between *SCN1A* and epilepsy in a subsequent paragraph.

There are more intricacies when considering complex febrile seizures. The general consensus is that children with complex febrile seizures have a slightly higher (4% to 8%) risk of having future epilepsy than the general population.[7] Children with focal signs have a 8% risk of developing later epilepsy. Among all single factors (eg, duration, number of seizures within 24 hours, and focality), focality has the highest risk; however, the combined factors are the most predictive (49%) of future epilepsy.[3] That risk is increased to greater than 20% in children with febrile status epilepticus.[4] Importantly, children who first present with a prolonged (> 15 minutes) febrile seizure are more likely to have recurrences of prolonged febrile seizures.[7] I believe it necessary to pursue both routine EEG and brain magnetic resonance imaging (MRI) for children with complex febrile seizures in order to uncover a potential anatomical seizure focus (see Table 3-2 for suggestions on emergency management of complex febrile seizures). If the results of these tests are normal, the child does not require evaluation by a child neurologist. However, for many families, seeing a neurologist for an initial evaluation can be reassuring so referral is at your discretion. The AAP does not recommend maintenance or emergency antiseizure medication for children with simple or complex febrile seizures.[1] Nonetheless, in the case of a child with a history of febrile status epilepticus, most child neurologists would prescribe emergency rectal diazepam to be used in seizures lasting 5 minutes or longer.

I do want to emphasize the importance of considering a child's overall developmental progress and family history when considering prognosis after any type of febrile seizure. If a child is developmentally abnormal prior to a febrile seizure, developmentally stalls or regresses following a febrile seizure, or has a parent with a history of both febrile seizures and epilepsy, the clinician needs to be concerned about a potential genetic epilepsy syndrome. A mutation in the *SCN1A* gene, a gene that encodes for a sodium channel receptor, is the most common known genetic mutation leading to epilepsy syndromes that include febrile seizures.[7,8] The phenotype of this mutation varies from only febrile seizures to Dravet syndrome, an epileptic encephalopathy. Once you are considering a potential genetic epilepsy, the child should be referred to a child neurologist for further evaluation.

Summary

My advice to pediatricians and parents on febrile seizures is that they are most often benign and do not significantly increase a child's risk of subsequent epilepsy. A child with simple febrile seizures does not warrant any additional investigation. Recurrent simple febrile seizures in children require child neurologist evaluation only when particular criteria are met. Children with complex febrile seizures should have both an outpatient EEG and an MRI to investigate for the possibility of an underlying seizure focus. Neurological referral for a complex febrile seizure is up to you and the child's parents. Lastly, if a child has a history of neurodevelopmental stagnation or regression following a febrile seizure, you should refer the child to a child neurologist for evaluation. The same is true for a child with a parent who had febrile seizures and subsequently developed epilepsy.

References

1. Steering Committee on Quality Improvement and Management, Subcommittee on Febrile Seizures, American Academy of Pediatrics. Febrile seizures: clinical practice guideline for long-term management of the child with simple febrile seizures. *Pediatrics.* 2008;121(6):1281-1286.
2. Marks WJ, Laxer KD. Semiology of temporal lobe seizures: value in lateralizing the seizure focus. *Epilepsia.* 1998;39(7):721-726.
3. Annegers JF, Hauser WA, Shirts SB, Kurland LT. Factors prognostic of unprovoked seizures after febrile convulsions. *N Engl J Med.* 1987:316(9):493-498.
4. Neligan A, Bell GS, Giavasi C, et al. Long-term risk of developing epilepsy after febrile seizures: a prospective cohort study. *Neurology.* 2012;78:1166-1170.
5. Hattori J, Ouchida M, Ono J, et al. A screening test for the prediction of Dravet syndrome before one year of age. *Epilepsia.* 2008;49(4):626-633.
6. Hirose S, Scheffer IE, Marini C, et al. *SCN1A* testing for epilepsy: application in clinical practice. *Epilepsia.* 2013;54(5):946-952.
7. Pavlidou E, Hagel C, Panteliadis C. Febrile seizures: recent developments and unanswered questions. *Childs Nerv System.* 2013;29(11):2011-2017.
8. Cross JH. Fever and fever-related epilepsies. *Epilepsia.* 2012;53(Suppl 4):3-8.

ARE THE BENIGN CHILDHOOD EPILEPSIES REALLY BENIGN?

Katherine S. Taub, MD

Telling a family that their child has epilepsy can be very difficult news to share. As the physician you try to reassure the parents, but hearing that their child may have to take a daily medicine and that extra safety precautions need to be taken, particularly around water because of the risk of drowning, makes it even harder for them to accept the diagnosis. However, during my training as a neurologist, I was taught that certain epilepsy syndromes were considered "benign" and thus an easier diagnosis to discuss with families. If you had to be diagnosed with one of the epilepsy syndromes, benign rolandic epilepsy (BRE) and childhood absence epilepsy (CAE) were "the best" epilepsy syndromes to have.

An epilepsy syndrome is considered benign based on the frequency of seizures, severity of seizures, and the overall prognosis. Children with BRE often have infrequent seizures thus decreasing the morbidity of the epilepsy syndrome and often preventing the need for daily medication. Even though children with CAE may have multiple seizures per day prior to treatment, the seizures are brief and often subtle. Absence seizures with behavioral arrest, eye fluttering, and lip smacking appear milder than generalized tonic-clonic seizures with whole body jerking, tongue biting, and incontinence, which most people imagine when they think of seizures. BRE and CAE are also considered more benign because of the potential to outgrow the syndrome in adolescence. Both types of epilepsy were also thought to not cause cognitive or psychosocial difficulties. However, recent long-term outcome studies of children with BRE and CAE show that they are not as "benign" as we used to think.

BRE, which is also known as benign epilepsy of childhood with central-temporal spikes, presents in children 5 to 12 years old. It is the most common epileptic syndrome with a prevalence of 23% to 24% among school-aged children with epilepsy.[1] The etiology of BRE is often not known but there is an associated hereditary predisposition, suggesting a genetic cause. The seizures are focal seizures involving the mouth and face, often causing drooling and slurred speech. Many

Licht DJ, Ryan NR, eds. *Curbside Consultation in Pediatric Neurology: 49 Clinical Questions* (pp 15-17).
© 2016 Taylor & Francis Group.

children have preservation of consciousness during the seizure thus being able to speak even though slurred and able to follow commands. The seizure may spread to become a focal motor seizure of the arm and hand, and may generalize. The majority of seizures occur in sleep but can occur during the day. The electroencephalogram (EEG) associated with BRE consists of central-temporal sharps from both the right and left hemisphere with a frontal dipole in a monopolar montage. Otherwise the EEG background is normal with no slowing.

BRE is considered benign since the seizures typically cease in adolescence, and it does not affect cognitive development. This epilepsy syndrome is not associated with structural brain abnormalities so imaging, such as magnetic resonance imaging (MRI), is not warranted. Owing to its benign nature with infrequent seizures and no cognitive deficits, antiepileptic medications are not recommended. Not treating the seizures does not lead to future seizures. In fact, children with BRE have the same risk of developing epilepsy in adulthood as the general population.

However, BRE is not benign from the perspective of the child who worries about when the next seizure will come. The child feels socially isolated, refusing to go to sleepovers for fear of having a seizure in front of his or her friends. Some of my patients have found the experience of a Todd's paralysis, unilateral weakness following a seizure, to be terrifying. Many parents would not characterize BRE as benign. They dread seeing their child with a facial droop slurring words as if he or she were having a stroke. Not all children with BRE have infrequent seizures, with 6% to 18% having frequent seizures.[1] For these children with frequent seizures and others traumatized by the seizures, I have prescribed antiepileptic medications such as Trileptal (oxcarbazepine) or Keppra (levetiracetam). I have also recommended Diastat (diazepam) as a rescue medication for patients whose focal seizures are either prolonged or develop into generalized tonic-clonic seizures lasting longer than 5 minutes.

There is an atypical course of BRE called atypical benign epilepsy of childhood or malignant rolandic-sylvian epilepsy (MRSE). These patients have oromotor deficits including facial weakness, dysarthria, and chewing or swallowing difficulties that may last for hours or continue intermittently over several days. The EEG of children with MRSE shows frequent seizures or status epilepticus arising from the rolandic area (motor strip) during these prolonged episodes. You should order an MRI of the brain for these patients to assess for structural brain abnormalities.[2] Other children thought to have BRE go on to develop electrical status epilepticus during slow sleep (ESES) in which at least 80% of their sleeping background consists of sharp and slow wave discharges on EEG. These children have language regression and severe behavior difficulties. Some children with BRE evolve into Landau-Kleffner syndrome, which is a catastrophic epilepsy syndrome associated with auditory agnosia and severe language regression. There is nothing benign in the clinical course of MRSE, ESES, or Landau-Kleffner syndrome.

CAE is a generalized epilepsy syndrome that develops in children from 5 to 10 years old that resolves in adolescence. You should inquire about a family history of generalized epilepsy. Absence seizures are often overlooked or misdiagnosed as daydreaming or attention difficulties. On EEG, the staring episodes correlate with a classic generalized 3-hertz spike and slow wave pattern. Since absence seizures are so subtle, they are considered to be milder. However, about 50% of patients may also develop generalized tonic-clonic seizures. It was not until studies like the Camfields' long-term outcome study of children with CAE that neurologists recognized that CAE was not as benign a syndrome as we had thought.[3]

The Camfields[3] compared the psychosocial challenges of patients with CAE to patients with another chronic childhood disease, juvenile rheumatoid arthritis (JRA), in all of Nova Scotia. Their study showed more psychosocial difficulties in patients with CAE, even those with seizure remission, compared to patients with JRA. Patients with CAE were less likely to graduate from high school and less likely to attend college. Later in life, adults with a prior diagnosis of CAE had higher unemployment rates and were less likely to hold upper level management positions. Forty percent of their cohort suffered from alcohol abuse. CAE patients were found to have a higher legal conviction rate than the general population of Nova Scotia. One-third of the CAE patients had unplanned pregnancies in their mid- to late teens. Other studies have also shown sleep difficulties, poor social adaption, and behavior problems in children with CAE. Neuropsychological testing can identify the specific areas of learning difficulties in at-risk children with CAE. The poor psychosocial skills, difficulty functioning in school, relationship troubles, and mental and behavioral health problems of patients with CAE make this epilepsy syndrome anything but benign.[4]

Perhaps doctors should not describe any epilepsy syndrome as benign as seen in the potentially complicated medical and social courses of patients with BRE and CAE. It is the responsibility of physicians to explain to their patients the spectrum of disease seen with their epilepsy syndromes. Parents should be educated about the learning and behavior disorders in children with these epilepsy syndromes in order to identify these difficulties early in a child's development and to seek extra help in school and professional behavioral therapy. Neuropsychological testing may also aid teachers in finding the most effective educational methods for children with epilepsy. Doctors should counsel their teens with epilepsy and their parents about the higher risks of sexual promiscuity, drug and alcohol abuse, and unemployment. We must all keep in mind that the term *benign* truly is in the eye of the beholder.

References

1. Kramer U. Atypical presentations of benign childhood epilepsy with centrotemporal spikes: a review. *J Child Neurol.* 2008;23:785.
2. Otsubo H. Malignant rolandic-sylvian epilepsy in children: diagnosis, treatment and outcomes. *Neurology.* 2001;57:590-596.
3. Camfield PR, Camfield CS. Epileptic syndromes in childhood: clinical features, outcomes and treatment. *Epilepsia.* 2002;43(Suppl 3):27-32.
4. Wirrell EC, Camfield CS, Camfield PR. Long-term psychosocial outcome in typical absence epilepsy. *Arch Pediatr Adolesc Med.* 1997;151(2):152-158.

DO SEIZURES CAUSE DEVELOPMENTAL DELAY? CAN TREATING THE SEIZURES HELP?

John R. Mytinger, MD

Most children with epilepsy are of normal intelligence and many excel in sports and academics. However, when compared to children without epilepsy, children with epilepsy are more likely to have developmental delay with cognitive, behavioral, and social dysfunction. These comorbidities and the epilepsy itself likely share a common etiology. Indeed, the underlying etiology of the epilepsy is a powerful predictor of developmental outcome. However, in some children, the epilepsy itself (ie, seizures) can variably contribute or be the major factor in determining the degree of comorbid developmental delay. There is mounting evidence to suggest that some seizures, and even spikes (see below), can negatively impact the developing brain and that early effective treatment can improve developmental outcome.

The Electroclinical Syndrome as a Predictor of Developmental Outcome

The International League Against Epilepsy (ILAE) defines an electroclinical syndrome as "a group of clinical entities that are reliably identified by a cluster of electroclinical characteristics." For example, childhood absence epilepsy is an electroclinical syndrome characterized clinically by absence seizures provoked by hyperventilation and electrographically by generalized 3-hertz spike-wave discharges on electroencephalogram (EEG). Traditionally, childhood absence epilepsy was considered one of several electroclinical syndromes associated with a "normal" developmental outcome. However, recent data find a strong association with attention deficit hyperactivity disorder and anxiety as well as cognitive and linguistic deficits. These difficulties can be present prior to the development of seizures and may well stem from the same underlying dysfunction ultimately

Licht DJ, Ryan NR, eds. *Curbside Consultation in Pediatric Neurology: 49 Clinical Questions* (pp 19-21).
© 2016 Taylor & Francis Group.

leading to seizures. That said, some data suggest that controlling seizures with medication can improve cognitive function. Thus, although many children with electroclinical syndromes like childhood absence epilepsy can do well, uncontrolled and frequent seizures likely have a negative effect on developmental outcome.

At the other end of the spectrum are those electroclinical syndromes associated with an epileptic encephalopathy. As defined by the ILAE, the term *epileptic encephalopathy* "embodies the notion that the epileptic activity itself may contribute to severe cognitive and behavioral impairments...." West syndrome, for example, is an electroclinical syndrome characterized by infantile spasms (a seizure type), developmental delay, and, classically, multifocal spikes and a chaotic, high-amplitude EEG background called hypsarrhythmia. While developmental outcomes in West syndrome are often poor, children with an unknown etiology (eg, normal brain magnetic resonance imaging and other investigations) and early successful treatment (remission of infantile spasms and hypsarrhythmia) can have a good developmental outcome. Yet, even for this group, delayed treatment is associated with lower developmental scores than those with early treatment. These findings suggest that ongoing infantile spasms and the associated EEG abnormalities negatively affect developmental outcome.

Spikes as a Contributor or Cause of Developmental Delay

A spike on an EEG represents the sudden synchronized discharge of a network of neurons—a finding that suggests an underlying predisposition for seizures. The question of whether spikes cause developmental delay is of great interest and some debate in the world of epilepsy. For most epilepsies, the prevention of seizures is a far more appropriate goal than the suppression of spikes. Spike suppression is often not feasible and may not be necessary to optimize developmental outcome. However, in several circumstances, frequent spikes are associated with developmental delay. Take "benign" epilepsy with centrotemporal spikes (BECTS) (better known as benign rolandic epilepsy), for example. In this electroclinical syndrome, spikes from the centrotemporal region are sleep activated and seizures commonly occur during sleep. Children with BECTS can have various degrees of dysfunction related to language and the degree of dysfunction may, in part, relate to spike frequency. Remission of spikes on EEG has been associated with normalization of language dysfunction. Some children with BECTS have infrequent nocturnal seizures and do not require treatment. Children with more frequent seizures, especially if they occur during the day, may require treatment. Those children with psychosocial dysfunction may benefit from seizure remission and spike suppression.

A much more severe example of how spikes may cause developmental delay is seen in children with the electroclinical syndromes of continuous spike wave of sleep (CSWS) and Landau-Kleffner syndrome. Both syndromes are associated with an epileptic encephalopathy, developmental regression, and electrical status epilepticus of sleep (ESES). ESES is an EEG pattern characterized by very frequent spikes during sleep. The percentage of 1-second bins during sleep that includes a spike-wave discharge can wax and wane from one night to the next but may exceed 85%. An EEG that includes sleep (typically performed overnight) is necessary to confirm the presence of ESES. In Landau-Kleffner syndrome, children most often present between the ages of 3 and 8 years with language regression and behavioral problems. The developmental regression for children with CSWS is not limited to language and typically includes other domains of development. Effective treatment of ESES can positively affect developmental outcome for some children.

The Impact of Seizures on the Developing Brain

Status epilepticus (traditionally defined as a seizure or seizures [without return to baseline] extending beyond 30 minutes) can result in neurodevelopmental deterioration due to hypoxic-ischemic changes and excitatory neurotoxicity. Younger children with status epilepticus appear to be at greatest risk. In addition, mounting evidence suggests that less-dramatic seizures, if uncontrolled, can negatively impact the developing brain. Roughly one-third of children with epilepsy have seizures that cannot be controlled with medication (ie, medically intractable epilepsy). Individuals with more frequent seizures are at risk of academic failure. In comparison to individuals with other seizure types, those with frequent convulsive seizures may be at greatest risk for cognitive dysfunction. The detrimental effect of delayed treatment on developmental outcome was already discussed previously for West syndrome. A delay in epilepsy surgery for children with medically refractory epilepsy is also associated with lower cognitive and developmental scores after surgery. This suggests that delays in the treatment of ongoing seizures expose the brain to unfavorable changes, and early effective treatment may prevent these changes. However, studies of a severe electroclinical syndrome like West syndrome and epilepsy surgery for medically intractable epilepsy are unable to clarify whether it is the duration of the epilepsy (earlier age of onset) or the ongoing seizures that have the greater influence on developmental outcome. Berg and colleagues[1] have addressed this uncertainty by comparing 2 groups of children: one with well-controlled epilepsy and the other with uncontrolled epilepsy. In very young children (epilepsy onset 0 to 3 years), developmental scores declined in the 3 years following diagnosis only in those with uncontrolled epilepsy but remained stable in those with well-controlled epilepsy—an effect that was confirmed when these children were evaluated 8 to 9 years later. These findings highlight the potentially positive impact of early and effective treatment for children with epilepsy in relation to ultimate developmental outcome.

Summary

Developmental delay is common in children with epilepsy. The epilepsy and associated developmental delay, if present, likely stem from a common etiology. However, multiple lines of evidence suggest that seizures (and for some, spikes) can negatively affect the developing brain. Early and effective treatment can positively impact developmental outcome.

Reference

1. Berg AT, Zelko FA, Levy SR, Testa FM. Age at onset of epilepsy, pharmacoresistance, and cognitive outcomes: a prospective cohort study. *Neurology.* 2012;79(13):1384-1391.

Suggested Readings

Hermann BP, Seidenberg M, Bell B. The neurodevelopmental impact of childhood onset temporal lobe epilepsy on brain structure and function and the risk of progressive cognitive effects. *Prog Brain Res.* 2002;135:429-438.

O'Callaghan FJ, Lux AL, Darke K, et al. The effect of lead time to treatment and of age of onset on developmental outcome at 4 years in infantile spasms: evidence from the United Kingdom Infantile Spasms Study. *Epilepsia.* 2011;52(7):1359-1364.

Sirén A, Kylliäinen A, Tenhunen M, et al. Beneficial effects of antiepileptic medication on absence seizures and cognitive functioning in children. *Epilepsy Behav.* 2007;11(1):85-91.

DOES EPILEPSY RUN IN FAMILIES?

Jason Coryell, MD, MS

When a family is sitting in front of me asking why their child has developed epilepsy, I typically pare it down to 2 main groups: genetic vs structural causes. (Disclaimer: The structural and genetic groups are not mutually exclusive, as can be illustrated in cases of tuberous sclerosis or lissencephaly.) While the 2 groups are of roughly equal size, there are multiple etiologies in each group, and the treatment, prognosis, and heritability of epilepsy may vary significantly depending on the underlying cause. The structural causes of epilepsy may be easier to tackle, as brain magnetic resonance imaging (or head computed tomography) often will demonstrate an identifiable lesion. Examples include a prior stroke (encephalomalacia), malformation of cortical development (eg, cortical dysplasia, schizencephaly), or tumor. The genetic causes of epilepsy are continuing to unfold, but include recognizable syndromes (eg, tuberous sclerosis), chromosomal abnormalities, and nonsyndromic single-gene disorders with epilepsy. There are also cases that are "presumed genetic" (also referred to as idiopathic epilepsy) that display more complex heritability (ie, multifactorial inheritance) with a limited understanding of gene-gene or gene-environment interactions.

The recurrence risk for other family members depends largely on the underlying etiology, and can range from < 1% with a new mutation up to 50% with autosomal-dominant conditions. Recurrence risk counseling can be narrowed when a specific diagnosis is obtained, often through the combination of a physical examination, classification of seizure types, family history, neuroimaging, and some preliminary lab testing (eg, chromosomal microarray). Multifactorial inheritance is the most common inheritance pattern in epilepsy, and commercial genetic testing is not available for most of these cases, making it difficult to estimate risk.

Licht DJ, Ryan NR, eds. *Curbside Consultation in Pediatric Neurology: 49 Clinical Questions* (pp 23-26).
© 2016 Taylor & Francis Group.

Recognizable Syndromes

When a syndrome is present, epilepsy often coexists with other neurologic and non-neurologic findings. Developmental delay/intellectual disability is a clue that the individual is not neurotypical; however, this is not a specific sign. Dysmorphic features, abnormal head circumference, abnormal pigmented macules/patches, or other systemic features can be more helpful in leading you toward a specific diagnosis. An affected parent or sibling with a history of seizures plus other findings often prompts me to collaborate with a clinical geneticist to look for additional minor or major findings that could narrow down the potential diagnoses. When epilepsy is the presenting sign, there may be few other systemic clues. For example, children with tuberous sclerosis may not have apparent hypopigmented areas ("ash leaf spots") or angiofibromas until later in childhood. Similarly, heart and renal findings may not be elicited unless renal ultrasound and echocardiogram are ordered. Syndromes may exhibit variable expressivity, and an affected parent with tuberous sclerosis may not have recognized signs of the disorder until a closer examination has been performed after the diagnosis of the child. Some syndromes may be diagnosed based on clinical features alone, while others require specific genetic testing.

Chromosomal Abnormalities

Chromosomal causes of epilepsy may include abnormal chromosome number (eg, trisomy 13), large deletions or duplications (eg, Wolf-Hirschhorn syndrome, due to deletion of chromosomal arm 4p), or chromosomal microdeletions (eg, DiGeorge syndrome). Standard karyotyping has been used to diagnose many of these conditions; however, comparative genomic hybridization (CGH) has improved our ability to find even smaller duplications and deletions by identifying copy number variants. CGH should be considered an early test if there are major/minor malformations, dysmorphic features, and/or intellectual disability in a child without a readily identifiable syndrome. Even in cases of epilepsy without other systemic findings, CGH has identified abnormalities in about 10%. An example of this is seen in 15q13.3 microdeletion, which can be associated with intellectual disability, autism, schizophrenia, or epilepsy.

Nonsyndromic Single-Gene Disorders

Specific epilepsy disorders are often defined based on seizure type, age of onset, and characteristic electroencephalogram (EEG) patterns. Some of these clinical syndromes have known genetic associations. Benign familial neonatal convulsions (BFNC) typically begin in the first week of life. This is an autosomal-dominant condition with high penetrance. The natural history is spontaneous resolution of seizures in the first few months of life, although seizure recurrence in later childhood or adulthood is 14%. The majority of cases of BFNC are attributable to potassium channel abnormalities. Dravet syndrome consists of the constellation of prolonged hemiconvulsive seizures in infancy, later myoclonic and/or absence seizures, ataxia, and acquired neurodevelopmental disability. Mutations in the sodium channel, voltage-gated, type I, alpha subunit (*SCN1A*) account for 70% to 80% of cases, most being sporadic rather than inherited. Genetic associations have been found with other epilepsy syndromes, although the sensitivity of genetic testing is variable. With autosomal-dominant nocturnal frontal lobe epilepsy, mutations in 2 different nicotinic acetylcholine receptors account for ~30% in patients with a positive family history. Progressive myoclonic epilepsies comprise a group of disorders with myoclonic seizures and developmental regression. These combined findings should prompt further systemic evaluation and genetic workup. There are additional genes for which commercial testing is possible; however, a comprehensive review of these conditions is beyond the scope of this chapter.

There can be significant inter- and intrafamilial variability in the severity of epilepsy. With *SCN1A* mutations, individuals may have the more severe Dravet phenotype, be seizure free, or have an intermediate phenotype of generalized epilepsy-febrile seizures plus, in which patients have febrile seizures beyond the age of 6 years or afebrile seizures (convulsive or absence). While difficult to prove, much of this variation is due to suspected environmental and genetic differences that modulate the expression of seizures.

Idiopathic Epilepsy

The genetic contribution to the remaining cases of nonsyndromic, nonlesional epilepsy is more complex. Twin studies have shown an increased concordance of epilepsy in monozygotic twins compared to dizygotic twins (44% vs 10%). Identical twins were also more likely to express epilepsy with the same seizure type than concordant fraternal twins. Although Berkovic reported greater concordance rates for generalized epilepsies compared to focal epilepsies (82% vs 36%), increased concordance in twins has been documented for focal-onset epilepsy in multiple populations as well. The concordance between subtypes of seizures (eg, temporal lobe epilepsy) was not statistically significant, reflecting that multiple seizures types can exist in the same family. Increased heritability has long been observed with idiopathic generalized epilepsy (IGE) at the family level, with many families showing dominant inheritance with reduced penetrance.

The umbrella term *IGE* includes common epilepsy syndromes such as childhood absence epilepsy (CAE) and juvenile myoclonic epilepsy (JME). In CAE, there are reported associations with different calcium channels in select families; however, it is unclear that any single gene is necessary for development of that seizure type. JME is a constellation of early-morning myoclonic, generalized tonic-clonic, and absence seizures, with typical EEG features, and commonly begins during adolescence. JME has been independently associated with abnormalities in gamma-aminobutyric acid receptors, chloride channels (*CLCN2*), as well as other genes and chromosomal loci not listed here. Conversely, many of these same genes have been associated with variable presentations (including different seizure types). For example, *CLCN2* has been associated with CAE, juvenile absence epilepsy, JME, and generalized tonic-clonic seizures upon awakening. More recent exome studies of unrelated individuals showed that there was no single variant with a large effect size (≥ 1%), suggesting that there are multiple susceptibility genes throughout the population with each accounting for a small fraction of individuals with epilepsy. The additive effect of multiple potential variants is not well understood.

Epilepsy due to a clear-cut Mendelian disorder accounts for a small percentage of all epilepsy cases. Online Mendelian Inheritance in Man currently lists nearly 600 associations with epilepsy, although this number includes rare syndromes and a rapidly expanding list of chromosomal variations reported in few families (added since the advent of microarrays). While a specific gene association eludes many cases, a suspected genetic predisposition remains in nearly half of epilepsy cases (often referred to as idiopathic epilepsy). Supportive data have come from twin studies, larger multiplex families, and genome-wide association studies. These have led to localization of chromosomal loci or specific genes that are more frequently associated with epilepsy phenotypes. These susceptibility genes may modulate an individual's risk for expressing seizures based on complex environmental interactions such as degree of expression during different developmental stages or interaction with other gene products.

Suggested Readings

Berkovic SF, Howell RA, Hay DA, Hopper JL. Epilepsies in twins: genetics of the major epilepsy syndromes. *Ann Neurol.* 1998;43(4):435-445.

Corey LA, Pellock JM, Kjeldsen MJ, Nakken KO. Importance of genetic factors in the occurrence of epilepsy syndrome type: a twin study. *Epilepsy Res.* 2011;97(1-2):103-111.

Cosette P. Channelopathies in juvenile myoclonic epilepsy. *Epilepsia.* 2010;51(Suppl 1):30-32.

Heinzen EL, Depondt C, Cavalleri GL, et al. Exome sequencing followed by large-scale genotyping fails to identify single rare variants of large effect in idiopathic generalized epilepsy. *Am J Hum Gen.* 2012;91(2):293-302.

Heinzen EL, Radtke RA, Urban TJ, et al. Rare deletions at 16p13.11 predispose to a diverse spectrum of sporadic epilepsy syndromes. *Am J Hum Genet.* 2010;86(5):707-718.

Mefford HC, Muhle H, Ostertag P, et al. Genome-wide copy number variation in epilepsy: novel susceptibility loci in idiopathic generalized and focal epilepsies. *PLoS Genet.* 2010;6(5):e1000962.

Mully JC, Mefford HC. Epilepsy and the new cytogenetics. *Epilepsia.* 2010;52(3):423-432.

ARE THERE ANY DIET CHANGES OR VITAMINS THAT MAY HELP A CHILD WITH EPILEPSY?

Adam L. Hartman, MD and Brian Masselink, MD

Yes! The concept that metabolism may affect seizures dates back to the time of Hippocrates and thus represents one of the oldest forms of antiseizure treatment.[1] Although the Internet is full of unconfirmed attestations about diet or vitamins improving or worsening seizures, altering metabolism to affect neuronal excitability remains a relatively underexplored topic in the scientific world. Diets such as the ketogenic diet or herbal supplements should be treated as equivalents to medicine in that they should be initiated only with the guidance of the child's neurologist. Such measures could interact or alter a current medical therapy, and like medicines, can have side effects.

Diets

Dietary treatments have been proven to be highly effective in some cases of epilepsy. There are multiple dietary options that are viable alternatives or adjuncts to modern medicines. The most commonly implemented forms of dietary therapy for seizures include the high-fat, low-carbohydrate ketogenic diet (which in our institution consists primarily of long-chain fatty acids), the medium-chain triglyceride ketogenic diet, the modified Atkins diet, and low glycemic index treatment (LGIT). Referral to a pediatric neurology center equipped to discuss dietary options with families is generally warranted if parents are interested.

Typically, dietary treatment of seizures is considered in 3 situations:

1. Glucose transporter type 1 (GLUT1) deficiency. Patients with mutations in GLUT1 cannot transport glucose effectively from the blood to the cerebrospinal fluid, resulting in neurological symptoms ranging from seizures to movement disorders. Because these patients cannot use glucose in the brain, the ketogenic diet provides fatty acids that are metabolized to acetyl

Licht DJ, Ryan NR, eds. *Curbside Consultation in Pediatric Neurology: 49 Clinical Questions* (pp 27-31).
© 2016 Taylor & Francis Group.

coenzyme A, which then is used as a substrate in the Krebs cycle for adenosine triphosphate (ATP) production. The ketogenic diet improves seizures and movement disorders in this condition, although developmental delays may persist.

2. Pyruvate dehydrogenase deficiency. The mechanism of the ketogenic diet's effect probably is the provision of alternate substrates, analogous to the situation in GLUT1 deficiency.

3. Medically intractable epilepsy. The definition of medically intractable epilepsy is somewhat fluid but most definitions encompass the concept that the patient's seizures are not adequately controlled by 2 or 3 medicines over a modest time frame. Certain epilepsy syndromes, such as Doose syndrome (ie, myoclonic astatic epilepsy), Dravet syndrome (ie, sodium channel, voltage-gated, type I, alpha subunit mutations), tuberous sclerosis complex (ie, *TSC1* and *2* mutations), and certain mitochondrial disorders (eg, complex I deficiency), may be particularly responsive to diet treatments. More recently, dietary treatments have even been used in the intensive care unit to treat cases of refractory status epilepticus. In contrast, ketogenic diets are contraindicated in pyruvate carboxylase deficiency, primary carnitine deficiency, beta-oxidation defects, and certain mitochondrial cytopathies because of either carbohydrate dependence or inability to metabolize fatty acids. The mechanism of all the diets is not entirely clear (discussed further later) but the diet is as efficacious as medicine in this context, frequently with fewer side effects.

As noted previously, the concept of dietary management of seizures dates back centuries and is based on the observation that fasting improves seizure control. Studies in humans and animal models have shown consistently that restriction of carbohydrates (which is common to all 4 diets) may have antiseizure effects but does not explain all the diets' effects. In particular, ketone bodies (ie, beta-hydroxybutyrate, acetoacetate, and acetone) affect neuronal excitability (ie, synaptic vesicle loading) and ion channels (ie, gamma-aminobutyric acid [GABA]$_A$, ATP-sensitive potassium), or neurotransmitters (ie, adenosine). The role of mitochondrial function, specific metabolism pathways (ie, mammalian target of rapamycin), and hormones (ie, brain-derived nerve growth factor or leptin) also are under current investigation. The type of fatty acid (ie, polyunsaturated fatty acids vs saturated fatty acids) does not appear to make a difference.

Practically speaking, ketogenic diets are implemented using a "ketogenic ratio" such as 3:1 or 4:1 (grams of fat to grams of combined protein and carbohydrate). The ketogenic diet may be started with or without an overnight fast; earlier responses are noted with a brief fast but long-term outcomes do not differ. Our institution implements an overnight fast in an inpatient setting (specifically, to monitor patients during the metabolic stress and because we frequently use an overnight fast to amplify the diet's effects during illnesses in the outpatient setting). Other institutions have initiated the diet successfully in the outpatient setting, as well. Education based on the diabetes model is offered during the initiation phase (ie, meal planning, sick day management). An example of a typical ketogenic diet menu is shown in Table 7-1. "Cheating" with occasional carbohydrate-rich foods may break the cycle of ketosis and lead to increased seizure frequency.

The modified Atkins diet and LGITs typically are implemented in the outpatient setting. The modified Atkins diet reduces carbohydrate intake but not to the same degree as in the ketogenic diet. Carbohydrates are generally restricted to 10 grams per day in children, without restriction in protein or calories. Increased fat intake is encouraged, and patients may achieve moderate ketosis. Adolescents frequently adhere to this regimen better than the traditional ketogenic diet (and families frequently join their teens on the diet, as well).

Unlike the other diets, the LGIT is not a high-fat diet. Carbohydrates are limited (40 to 60 grams per day), but they are restricted to those foods with a glycemic index (ie, levels compared to the rise in blood sugar compared to glucose) of less than 50.

Table 7-1
Typical Ketogenic Diet Menu

- Breakfast: eggs and cheese
- Lunch: chicken with mayonnaise and avocado
- Dinner: beef with cheese, butter, and broccoli
- Snack: cheesecake

Table 7-2
Website Resources for Information on the Ketogenic Diet

- www.charliefoundation.org
- www.epilepsy.com/learn/treating-seizures-and-epilepsy/dietary-therapies/ketogenic-diet
- www.ilae.org/Commission/medther/keto-index.cfm
- www.matthewsfriends.org

For all diets, the involvement of a dietician familiar with its specifics is critical. Most would argue it is more important to have a dietician who can supervise the diet than a physician. Potential side effects of ketogenic diets include metabolic acidosis, hypoglycemia, constipation, and exacerbation of gastroesophageal reflux. Long-term effects may include constipation (with long-chain fatty acid diets), diarrhea (with medium-chain triglyceride diets), growth restriction, increased long bone fracture susceptibility, dyslipidemia, nephrolithiasis, and deficiency of calcium, vitamin D, or selenium. Improvement can be seen in seizure reduction within a few weeks, but parents should be aware of a minimum commitment of a few months to test true efficacy. Typically, responsive patients may continue the diet for 2 years before a weaning attempt.

Are diets effective? Multiple case series and meta-analyses both of retrospective and prospective studies have shown the ketogenic diet's efficacy. In a randomized controlled study, the ketogenic diet also was found to be more effective than watchful waiting.[2] The modified Atkins diet and LGIT have similar (possibly slightly lower) efficacy in case series, as well.

Given the multiple options, how can a family decide? It is best to refer to a pediatric neurology center with experience using these diets for further information and evaluation. Parents can be guided to certain websites (Table 7-2) or books for more information.

Vitamins

The most familiar example of vitamin treatment for epilepsy is vitamin B_6 (pyridoxine) dependency.[3] Seizures in the disorder (including status epilepticus) typically occur in early infancy but have been reported later in childhood, as well. Other findings include hypothermia and dystonia. Developmental delays and other encephalopathic findings may be seen. Many patients with this disorder do not have low blood levels of B_6 but rather seizures (and the electroencephalogram [EEG]) improve with B_6 supplementation. Initially, B_6 can be given intravenously (with concomitant cardiorespiratory and EEG monitoring) but the lack of a response on EEG usually is followed by genetic testing (aldehyde dehydrogenase 7 family, member A1, the gene that encodes antiquitin), measurement of pipecolic acid levels, and a trial of oral medication that typically lasts 3 to 6 weeks. If testing indicates B_6 dependency, treatment is lifelong. Similar syndromes have been described for pyridoxal phosphate (the biologically active form of pyridoxine) and folinic acid. Vitamins (eg, vitamin C or E) also may be prescribed as part of a "mitochondrial cocktail" to bypass metabolic blocks in enzymes or electron transport chain function.

Other Herbs and Supplements

Supplemental products are sometimes commonly used remedies that often lack sufficient data to prove efficacy, lack regulation and standardization of manufacturing, and may cause unintended harm. In general, it is wise to specifically ask about the use of herbs or traditional medicines. Herbal remedies may not be initially disclosed by the family but may be influencing seizure presentation by either lowering seizure threshold or interfering with hepatic metabolism. Examples include gingko, a cytochrome P450 2C19-inducer that can reduce levels of valproate or phenytoin. Gingko also can have proconvulsant effects via GABA-ergic inhibition. Some folk remedies may include undisclosed medications, including anticonvulsant medications like phenytoin.

Common supplements that are considered possibly beneficial with seizures are kava, valerian, and melatonin. Kava is an herbal remedy whose mechanism of action includes calcium channel inhibition and weak sodium channel blocking. It has gained popularity as an anxiolytic and there are anecdotal reports of efficacy in epilepsy. Clinical studies, however, are lacking.

Valerian root has been used as an anticonvulsant for centuries, and is commonly used today to help aid sleep. While the chemical makeup of the plant varies with age and growing conditions, one component is isovaleric acid, which is structurally analogous to valproic acid. Despite the similarity with the modern anticonvulsant, valerian root does not have proven clinical efficacy.

Melatonin has been studied as an adjuvant medication in epilepsy. A Cochrane review in 2012 considered 4 randomized, double-blind, placebo-controlled trials investigating melatonin and concluded there were insufficient data to recommend melatonin for the treatment of epilepsy. Neither seizure control nor quality of life was improved. One good resource for complementary and alternative medicines is the National Center for Complementary and Integrative Health (https://nccih.nih.gov/).

Marijuana-Derived Cannabinoid Products

Another option that has been discussed widely in the media is marijuana-derived cannabinoid products. Examples include preparations containing cannabidiol and other substances that act on cannabinoid receptors. The safety of these products has not been clearly defined. The efficacy of these chemicals has not been studied in rigorously designed trials as of this writing (a number of industry-sponsored trials are underway). One problem is that different products contain varying concentrations of active ingredients, making comparisons very difficult. A number of legal issues (including debates on state vs federal regulations) still exist. Data on this topic are presented frequently, so consultation with current literature is recommended before discussing this class of compounds with families.

References

1. Kossoff EH, Hartman AL. Ketogenic diets: new advances for metabolism-based therapies. *Curr Opin Neurol.* 2012;25(2):173-178.
2. Neal EG, Chaffe H, Schwartz RH, et al. The ketogenic diet for the treatment of childhood epilepsy: a randomised controlled trial. *Lancet Neurol.* 2008;7(6):500-506.
3. Pearl PL. New treatment paradigms in neonatal metabolic epilepsies. *J Inherit Metab Dis.* 2009;32(2):204-213.

QUESTION

Do Children "Outgrow" Epilepsy?

Emily A. Gertsch, MD, MPH and Kelly Knupp, MD

A diagnosis of epilepsy during childhood can be difficult for parents given the sometimes frightening nature of seizures, treatments, and social implications associated with epilepsy. It then follows that a natural question asked of the treating physician is, "Will my child outgrow this condition?" In essence, parents who pose this question are asking if their child will be able to live a life free of seizures and their treatments. While the answer is complex and dependent on many variables, this chapter will attempt to address some of these variables and identify risk factors that guide the physician in identifying those children who will be seizure free and those who have the greatest likelihood of achieving a life without antiseizure medications. There are many factors to consider when attempting to predict seizure outcome, including the type of seizure, epilepsy syndrome, etiology, individual patient characteristics, and patient electroencephalogram (EEG) or imaging results (Table 8-1). We will discuss a few of these factors thought to be most helpful in determining whether a child is likely to "outgrow" his or her epilepsy.

One of the most important factors in determining which children are most likely to achieve complete seizure remission off medications is the underlying etiology. It is thus important to begin our discussion by differentiating the 3 fundamental seizure classifications as previously defined by the International League Against Epilepsy: remote symptomatic, cryptogenic, and idiopathic. It is important to note that the seizure classification was recently updated to categorize seizures as genetic, structural-metabolic, or unknown, rather than the above-mentioned classification scheme. However, because the new classification system is less familiar to treating physicians and previous studies examining outcomes in children with epilepsy rely on the older system, we will refer to the older classification scheme for the purposes of our discussion.

Remote symptomatic epilepsy occurs in individuals without an immediate cause but with an identifiable previous brain injury or static encephalopathy (ie, cerebral palsy). Cryptogenic epilepsy affects individuals with seemingly normal development and cognition without a clear

Licht DJ, Ryan NR, eds. *Curbside Consultation in Pediatric Neurology: 49 Clinical Questions* (pp 33-36).
© 2016 Taylor & Francis Group.

Table 8-1
Risk Factors to Consider for Predicting Outcome

- Seizure classification or etiology
- Epilepsy syndrome
- Age at onset
- EEG pattern
- Brain imaging results
- Presence or absence of neurologic deficits on examination
- Response to antiseizure medication
- Temporal pattern of seizures
- Duration of seizures
- Seizure frequency
- History of febrile seizures

---

etiology. Idiopathic epilepsy encompasses the presumed genetic epilepsies, including benign rolandic epilepsy, childhood absence epilepsy, and juvenile myoclonic epilepsy, to name a few of the more commonly diagnosed epilepsies. Idiopathic epilepsy is often grouped with cryptogenic epilepsy in that both classifications lack an identifiable etiology. However, as genetic testing for various epilepsy syndromes becomes more sophisticated and commonly used, we will encounter more children with identifiable genetic epilepsies that are each associated with its own favorable or unfavorable risk in terms of achieving remission, which will become clearer as we continue to learn more about each of these genetic syndromes.

Children with remote symptomatic epilepsy associated with a congenital malformation, motor handicap, prior neurologic insult, or other identifiable neurologic abnormality are less likely to achieve seizure freedom off medications. Several studies show an increased risk for ongoing seizures in this group of patients as compared to patients with cryptogenic or idiopathic epilepsy. One study showed that 42% of children with neurologic abnormalities who have remote symptomatic epilepsy experienced seizure recurrence within 2 years after withdrawal of antiseizure medications, as opposed to 26% of children with cryptogenic epilepsy. Other studies have shown similar results, with children who have remote symptomatic epilepsy being approximately 1.5 times more likely than children with cryptogenic epilepsy to have seizure recurrence when medications are discontinued.[1]

Age of seizure onset has been shown to be predictive in determining which children are most likely to achieve seizure remission. Children whose initial seizure occurs before adolescence have a better prognosis for achieving seizure freedom. While there is some controversy about the prognosis of children who have a very early age of onset (less than 2 years of age), it is clear that patients with remote symptomatic epilepsy who experience their first seizure within the first 2 years of life do have a lower chance of entering remission.[1] Results have been conflicting when studying the outcomes of children with cryptogenic or idiopathic epilepsy who have very early age of onset.

The EEG has been useful in some cases to determine who is most likely to be successful in discontinuing antiseizure medications without seizure recurrence. EEG is important in identifying specific patterns seen in certain epilepsy syndromes, such as benign rolandic epilepsy (benign epilepsy with central temporal spikes), childhood absence epilepsy, and juvenile myoclonic epilepsy, each of which is associated with its own risk of relapse after medication withdrawal. In addition,

---

Table 8-2
Factors Not Associated With Outcome

- Seizure frequency prior to treatment
- Medication used
- Family history of seizures
- Number of seizures
- Type of seizures
- Duration of epilepsy

---

studies show that interictal EEG abnormalities, particularly epileptiform but also nonepileptiform abnormalities, seen prior to discontinuing antiseizure medications are associated with a decreased chance of achieving remission only in children with cryptogenic epilepsy.[1] EEG findings do not appear to be predictive of outcome in children with remote symptomatic epilepsy. It is unclear whether EEG changes between the onset of seizures and time of medication withdrawal are associated with risk of relapse.

Other factors have been found to have no association with relapse risk in children who discontinue antiseizure medications (Table 8-2). These factors include family history of epilepsy, initial seizure frequency, duration of epilepsy, number of seizures, and medication used for treatment.[1,2] Seizure type has also generally not been predictive of outcome, although children who have multiple seizure types typically are less likely to be seizure free.

However, one should not think about seizure control alone; there are other factors when considering the long-term consequences of childhood epilepsy. It is important to note that all children with epilepsy are at risk of having poor social, cognitive, and behavioral outcomes irrespective of eventual seizure control either with or without medications. Studies show that measures of learning, memory span, attention, and behavior are worse among school-age children with epilepsy as compared to healthy peers.[3] In addition, patients with idiopathic generalized epilepsy continue to have social difficulties into adulthood, including lower rates of high school completion and higher rates of unemployment, unplanned pregnancy, legal conviction, psychiatric diagnosis, and living alone.[4] The mechanism for these poor outcomes is unclear, but it is hypothesized that pre-existing neurodevelopmental abnormalities, epileptogenesis, genetic susceptibility, and environmental factors may be responsible. It is important for clinicians and parents to recognize these potential risks even after seizure freedom has been achieved in order to use appropriate measures for prevention and intervention.

Considering many of these factors, the majority of patients with childhood-onset epilepsy who initially achieve seizure control will achieve long-term remission. Treating physicians may use this information as a guide in discussing with families the likely outcome of their child in regard to the likelihood of seizure freedom off medications. As always, it is important to remember each patient is a unique individual with many variables to consider when contemplating the withdrawal of antiseizure medications. The decision to discontinue treatment for a child whose seizures are well controlled on an antiseizure regimen requires an open conversation with the family about the risks and benefits of withdrawing medications so the patient and family can be involved in an informed decision-making process.

References

1. Tsur VG, O'Dell C, Shinnar S. Initiation and discontinuation of antiepileptic drugs. In: Wyllie E, Cascino GD, Gidal BE, Goodkin HP, eds. *Wyllie's Treatment of Epilepsy: Principles and Practice.* 5th ed. Philadelphia, PA: Lippincott Williams & Wilkins; 2011:527-539.
2. Berg AT, Testa FM, Levy SR. Complete remission in nonsyndromic childhood-onset epilepsy. *Ann Neurol.* 2011;70(4):566-573.
3. Seneviratne U, Cook M, D'Souza W. The prognosis of idiopathic generalized epilepsy. *Epilepsia.* 2012;53(12):2079-2090.
4. Camfield P, Camfield C. Idiopathic generalized epilepsy with generalized tonic-clonic seizures (IGE-GTC): a population-based cohort with >20 year follow up for medical and social outcome. *Epilepsy Behav.* 2010;18(1-2):61-63.

QUESTION

WHAT ARE COMMON SIDE EFFECTS OF ANTISEIZURE MEDICATIONS?

Laufey Yr Sigurdardottir, MD

Side Effects of Antiepileptic Drugs

Antiepileptic drugs (AEDs) decrease neuronal excitability by altering sodium or calcium ion channel function, reducing glutamate-induced excitation, or increasing gamma-aminobutyric acid (GABA)-ergic inhibition. The oldest agents such as phenobarbital (PHB) and phenytoin (PHT) have a potent antiseizure effect but fairly prominent side effects while the newer, third-generation agents have been engineered to keep the desired antiseizure effect at its peak but to decrease bothersome side effects as well as dangerous adverse effects (AEs) that can potentially be fatal. It is very important for every clinician who manages patients with epilepsy to have a basic understanding of AEs. Many of them can be prevented or minimized with prompt recognition and treatment.

AEDs are the group of drugs most frequently associated with fatal drug reactions. One of the major challenges of AED therapy is preventing and managing AEs during treatment.

To maximize therapeutic success, it is key to recognize the type of seizure and/or the epileptic syndrome at hand. This will help the clinician optimize drug selection and assist in preventing the unfavorable interaction seen with certain drug types when used in specific seizure types or epilepsy syndromes.

AEs can be classified as dose-related AEs and idiosyncratic AEs. Table 9-1 lists AEs of AEDs.

Licht DJ, Ryan NR, eds. *Curbside Consultation in Pediatric Neurology: 49 Clinical Questions* (pp 37-42).
© 2016 Taylor & Francis Group.

Table 9-1
Adverse Effects of Antiepileptic Drugs

Antiepileptic Drug	Drug Type	Dose-Dependent Adverse Effects	Idiosyncratic Adverse Effects
Phenobarbital[a] +	Barbiturate	Sedation, hyperactivity in children	Rash, blood dyscrasias, hepatitis
Phenytoin[a] +	Hydantoin	Nystagmus, ataxia, drowsiness	Rash, serum sickness, hepatitis, blood dyscrasias
Valproic acid –	Fatty acid	Tremor, weight gain, hair loss	Blood dyscrasias, pancreatitis, hepatitis
Oxcarbazepine[a] +	Carboxamides	Hyponatremia, dizziness, somnolence, headache	Rash, blood dyscrasias
Carbamazepine[a] +	Carboxamides	Sedation, weight gain, nystagmus, GI upset	Rash, blood dyscrasias
Lamotrigine[a] +	Triazines	Ataxia, somnolence, headache	Rash, hepatic failure (rare)
Topiramate +	Fructose derivative	Cognitive slowing, weight loss, fatigue, renal stones	Rash
Levetiracetam	Pyrrolidines	Sedation, fatigue, dizziness	Psychiatric disturbances, blood dyscrasias
Zonisamide[a]	Sulfonamide	Somnolence, ataxia, anorexia	Rash, blood dyscrasias, renal failure
Ethosuximide	Succinimide	GI distress, hyponatremia, dizziness	Rash, hepatitis, blood dyscrasias
Vigabatrin +	Fatty acid	Sedation, depression, psychiatric symptoms	Visual field loss
Rufinamide	Unknown	Diplopia, dizziness, headache, somnolence, nausea	–
Lacosamide	Functionalized amino acid	Dizziness, suicidal ideation, arrhythmia	–

(continued)

Table 9-1 (continued)
Adverse Effects of Antiepileptic Drugs

Antiepileptic Drug	Drug Type	Dose-Dependent Adverse Effects	Idiosyncratic Adverse Effects
Gabapentin	GABA analog	Sleepiness, dizziness, ataxia, weight gain	Rash (rare)
Tiagabine	Fatty acid	Dizziness, somnolence, headache	Rare
Clonazepam	Benzodiazepine	Ataxia, incoordination, irritability	Rare (hematologic, hepatic)
Diazepam	Benzodiazepine	Ataxia, incoordination, irritability	Rare (hematologic, hepatic)
Clobazam	Benzodiazepine	Ataxia, incoordination, irritability	Rare (hematologic, hepatic)
Felbamate[a]	Carbamate	GI distress, headache, insomnia, weight loss	Rash, marrow suppression, hepatic failure
Stiripentol –	Aromatic allylic alcohol	GI distress	–
Pregabalin	GABA analog	Dizziness, somnolence, dry mouth, edema, weight gain	Rare
Acetazolamide	Sulfonamide	Lethargy, paresthesias, dizziness, nausea	Aplastic anemia
Sulthiame	Sulfonamide	Hyperpnea, headache, somnolence, ataxia	Rash

[a]Aromatic antiepileptic drug.

GI: gastrointestinal; GABA: gamma-aminobutyric acid; +: enzyme-inducing agent; –: enzyme inhibitor.

Dose-Related Adverse Effects

Most dose-related AEs are predictable based on the drug's pharmacologic properties. They can often be managed by decreasing the daily dose or slowing the upward titration of the agent. These events will usually not require discontinuation of therapy.

Risk factors for dose-related AEs include the following:

- Presence of other diseases, such as liver or kidney failure, which should always be considered both when choosing an agent and when dosing is considered

- Large starting doses and/or steep upward titration

- Polypharmacy, which increases the incidence of dose-related AEs and the risk of potential drug toxicity

The most common dose-related AEs relate to several anatomical systems: central nervous system, gastrointestinal system, genitourinary system, and skin. Various central nervous system symptoms such as cognitive and/or behavioral problems, headaches, dizziness, and movement disorders are collectively the most common AEs, with gastrointestinal symptoms such as nausea, vomiting, abdominal pain, constipation, or diarrhea being the second most common. Less frequent symptoms are fever, rash, and possible kidney stones.

Effective AED management depends on medication compliance, which is often jeopardized because of behavioral/cognitive side effects in the young patient. The incidence of behavioral-related AEs are related to the age of the patient, epilepsy type, predisposing learning disability, and/or previous behavioral/psychiatric disorders. The spectrum of behavioral/psychiatric symptoms related to AED therapy includes ill-defined symptoms such as somnolence, asthenia, and lethargy. Mood imbalance with anxiety, emotional lability, and/or frank depression are more concerning, and self-control difficulties with aggression, agitation, and challenging behavior can limit the use of certain AEDs despite promising seizure control.

Parents of young children with epilepsy are understandably worried about possible AEs of the AEDs on their behavior or cognition. The magnitude of AED-related cognitive slowing is generally mild to none in monotherapy with daily doses within normal ranges. Topiramate (TPX) is the AED that has been shown to carry the highest incidence of AEs including poor attention, memory difficulties, dysphasia, and possible cognitive slowing. Up to 50% of treated patients report some AEs associated with TPX treatment. Levetiracetam (LEV) is another agent with up to 30% incidence of behavioral AEs. This medication has not, however, been reported to cause cognitive slowing. Some AEDs (ie, valproic acid [VPA], lamotrigine [LTG]) have beneficial behavioral/psychiatric effects and are used for mood stabilization as well as for their antiepileptic effect. PHB is an old and effective AED but has been found to cause cognitive slowing, which seems to be at least in part reversible. This finding has limited the use of PHB in infants and young children for that reason.

Idiosyncratic Adverse Effects

Idiosyncratic AEs are sporadic and occur irrespective of dosage. Most individuals will not get these reactions irrespective of being on high doses for prolonged periods of time. Others seem to be susceptible to these events, and knowing such patient characteristics helps the clinician to identify "at-risk" individuals. It is necessary to weigh the benefits and risks of therapy with the patient/family.

The risk factors for idiosyncratic AEs include the following:

- Genetic predisposition, young age of patient, other diseases, such as autoimmune diseases and certain metabolic disorders (discussed below), AED type (ie, CYP450/UGT enzyme-inducing medication and aromatic AEDs are more likely to cause idiosyncratic reactions than other types of AEDs) and previous history of hypersensitivity reactions.

- Cytochrome P-450 isoenzyme (CYP450)-inducing AEDs include carbamazepine (CBZ), PHT, and PHB.

- Uridine 5'-diphospho (UDP)-glucuronosyltransferase (UGT)-inducing AEDs include CBZ, PHT, PHB, and VPA.

- Aromatic AEDs include LTG, PHT, PHB, CBZ, oxcarbazepine (OXC), felbamate (FEL), and zonisamide (ZNS).

The most common manifestations of an idiosyncratic reaction are as follows:

- Cutaneous, with severity ranging from a mild self-limiting maculopapular/morbilliform rash, to the more severe Stevens-Johnson syndrome (< 10% skin surface involvement) to the life-threatening toxic epidermal necrolysis (> 30% skin surface involvement), which carries a 30% mortality. Systemic involvement is frequently seen with fever, arthralgia/arthritis, and eosinophilia.

- Hematologic, with bone marrow suppression resulting in aplastic anemia or selective suppression of single cell lines (thrombocytopenia, anemia).

- Gastrointestinal, with hepatotoxicity, ranging from elevated transaminases without any signs of altered hepatic function to life-threatening fulminant liver necrosis. Pancreatitis is less common but should always be considered in patients on AEDs who are complaining of abdominal pain with/without vomiting.

Three main pathogenetic mechanisms are seen in idiosyncratic AEs: direct cytotoxicity, immune-mediated hypersensitivity reactions, and off-target pharmacology.

- Direct cytotoxicity: The best example of direct cytotoxicity is the hepatotoxicity seen with VPA therapy. This drug reaction is thought to be due to the direct cytotoxic effect of 2 VPA metabolites on the liver without an intermediate effect from the immune system. One of these metabolites is more prominent in infants and could explain the reason for the increased risk of hepatic failure in infants taking VPA. Metabolic diseases such as urea cycle disorders, organic acidurias, multiple carboxylase deficiency, respiratory chain dysfunction, pyruvate dehydrogenase deficiency, and pyruvate carboxylase deficiency all predispose to VPA-induced hepatotoxicity as do spinocerebellar ataxias, Friedreich ataxia, Alpers-Huttenlocher disease, and Lafora body disease.

- Immune-mediated hypersensitivity reaction: This involves abnormal responses within the humoral or cell-mediated immune system. The drug itself or one of its metabolites binds to and modifies a macromolecule that triggers an immune response. An example of this type of a reaction occurs when VPA and LTG are taken simultaneously. VPA inhibits the main clearance pathway of LTG, glucuronidation, which forces LTG to use the alternate CYP-mediated pathway. The metabolites formed through this pathway seem to provoke an immune response resulting in a hypersensitivity reaction and rash.

- Off-target pharmacology: This occurs when a drug interacts directly with a system other than that for which it is intended. A good example of this type of idiosyncratic reaction is AED-induced dyskinesia, TPX-induced glaucoma, or VPA-induced Fanconi syndrome.

Summary

AED-related AEs are undeniable, but having basic knowledge of the different types of AEs and knowing who is at risk and what epilepsy type you are treating will help limit the frequency of AEs and help clinicians recognize AEs when they occur so they treat them appropriately. The patient's risk of ongoing seizures will by far outweigh the risk of AEs if the drug of choice is selected after weighing the patient's epilepsy type and patient characteristics.

Suggested Readings

Eddy CM, Rickards HE, Cavanna AE. Behavioral adverse effects of antiepileptic drugs in epilepsy. *J Clin Psychopharmaocol.* 2012;32(3):362-375.

Guerrini R, Zaccara G, la Marca G, Rosati A. Safety and tolerability of antiepileptic drug treatment in children with epilepsy. *Drug Saf.* 2012;35(7):519-533.

Mikati MA. Seizures in childhood. In: Kliegman RM, Behrman RE, Jenson HB, Stanton BF, eds. *Nelson Textbook of Pediatrics.* 19th ed. Philadelphia, PA: Saunders/Elsevier Inc; 2011:2013-2039.

Park SP, Kwon SH. Cognitive effects of antiepileptic drugs. *J Clin Neurol.* 2008;4(3):99-106.

Wilfong A. Overview of the treatment of seizures and epileptic syndromes in children. Available at http://www.uptodate.com/contents/overview-of-the-treatment-of-seizures-and-epileptic-syndromes-in-children. Accessed March 20, 2015.

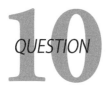

WHEN IS EPILEPSY CONSIDERED "REFRACTORY"? WHAT HAPPENS NEXT?

Karen L. Skjei, MD

Refractory epilepsy is a major source of morbidity and mortality in children. It is typically defined as inadequate seizure control despite trials of 2 appropriately chosen antiepileptic drugs (AEDs) at maximally tolerated doses. After 2 AED trials fail for lack of efficacy, the probability of achieving complete seizure control with a third AED is as low as 5% to 10%. The chance of complete seizure control diminishes further with each successive AED failure.[1]

In cases of refractory epilepsy, the first question you should consider should be, "Is this really epilepsy?" Misdiagnosis of nonepileptic events as seizures is common. Syncope, "pseudo-seizures," and migraine are all frequent diagnoses in pediatric populations and can be confused with epileptic events. Up to a quarter of patients diagnosed with refractory seizures may suffer from nonepileptic events.[2] Misdiagnoses are most often due to inaccurate history-taking and/or misinterpretation of electroencephalograms (EEGs). The National Association of Epilepsy Centers guidelines recommend referral to an epilepsy specialty center for more intensive EEG monitoring for patients whose events remain uncontrolled after 1 year, or for refractory patients. Long-term inpatient video-EEG monitoring (LTM) provides several advantages to routine EEGs in the evaluation of medically refractory epilepsy. The inpatient setting provides a safe environment for tapering and/ or withdrawal of AEDs. LTM also allows for extension of the recording until event(s) have been recorded. Several studies have shown ictal yields of approximately 70% to 85% in patients admitted to specialized epilepsy centers for LTM, leading to changes in diagnosis and management in up to 70% of patients. If the initial admission fails to provide a diagnosis, readmissions can have a yield of up to 40%.

When the diagnosis of epilepsy is confirmed, the next question to ask is, "Is the epilepsy truly refractory?" Seizures may be wrongly described as treatment resistant if trials of optimal first-line drugs are not attempted, inadequate doses are administered, or appropriate doses are given but for insufficient duration. Furthermore, certain AEDs can actually precipitate or worsen certain

Licht DJ, Ryan NR, eds. *Curbside Consultation in Pediatric Neurology: 49 Clinical Questions* (pp 43-49).
© 2016 Taylor & Francis Group.

seizure types. Medication noncompliance, sleep deprivation, recreational drug use, and alcohol can be contributory factors.

Once intractability has been convincingly established, an important question to consider is, "Is there an underlying etiology that may guide medical/surgical treatment decisions?" Refractory epilepsy can be associated with a wide variety of etiologies, from developmental brain anomalies to genetic/metabolic and autoimmune/inflammatory disorders (Table 10-1). Children with refractory epilepsy along with failure to thrive, episodes of vomiting and lethargy, or mental retardation should receive genetic and/or metabolic evaluation. Abnormalities in the neurologic exam, including dysmorphisms or abnormalities of head circumference, tone, vision, or hearing, merit scrutiny. A strong family history of seizures, mental retardation, or early/unexplained death should prompt similar evaluation.

Genetic disorders associated with refractory epilepsy include tuberous sclerosis complex, Angelman syndrome, trisomies (21, 13), the progressive myoclonic epilepsies, and mutations in ion channel genes, such as sodium channel, voltage-gated, type I, alpha subunit (*SCN1A*). *SCN1A* mutations can produce a wide spectrum of epilepsy phenotypes, from isolated febrile seizures to severe myoclonic epilepsy of infancy (Dravet syndrome). Genetic tests, including karyotype, microarrays, and testing for specific genes (targeted fluorescence in situ hybridization vs gene sequencing) are available at many commercial labs and should be tailored to the patient. *SCN1A* testing must be considered for potential surgical candidates, as epilepsy surgery is unsuccessful in these individuals, even in cases where magnetic resonance imaging (MRI) and EEG appear to localize seizure onset.[3]

Nearly 200 inborn errors of metabolism (IEM) have also been associated with seizures and epilepsy, many of which are resistant to treatment with standard AEDs.[2] While the individual diseases are rare, the collective incidence of IEM is estimated at 1 in 800 to 2500 births. Newborn screening programs increase detection of IEM, but are not comprehensive. Every child with unexplained refractory epilepsy should receive a basic metabolic screen including blood glucose, ammonia, acid base status, lactate, and urinary ketones. Depending on clinical presentation, this can be expanded as indicated to include the studies listed in Table 10-2.

Inflammatory/autoimmune causes such as Rasmussen syndrome or systemic lupus erythematosus should also be considered in cases of treatment-resistant seizures, especially in the context of known or suspected systemic autoimmune disorders or in association with neuropsychiatric manifestations such as psychosis or subacute encephalopathy. Rheumatologic screening labs such as complete blood count (CBC) with differential, erythrocyte sedimentation rate (ESR), C-reactive protein (CRP), thyroid function tests, rheumatoid factor, antinuclear antibodies (ANA) panel, antiphospholipid Ab, anticardiolipin Ab, angiotensin-converting enzyme (ACE), and antineutrophil cytoplasmic antibody (ANCA) should be considered. Cerebrospinal fluid (CSF) studies should include cell count with differential, total protein, immunoglobulin (Ig) G index, oligoclonal bands, and cytology. If paraneoplastic studies are sent, expanded markers—including voltage-gated potassium channel (VGKC) complex, N-methyl D-aspartate receptor antibody (NMDA R Ab), α-amino-3-hydroxy-5-methyl-4-isoxazolepropionic acid receptor (AMPA R), and gamma-aminobutyric acid B receptor (GABA-B R), should be obtained. Finally, in the proper clinical context, empiric trials of anti-inflammatory drugs such as adrenocorticotropic hormone (ACTH), steroids, intravenous immunoglobulin (IVIG), and/or plasma exchange may be indicated.

Once it is clear that the epilepsy is refractory and underlying, treatable genetic, metabolic, and autoimmune/inflammatory etiologies have been ruled out, the next question to consider is, "Is this child a potential candidate for epilepsy surgery?" Epilepsy surgery is the only intervention that has the potential to "cure" refractory seizures. Surgical success rates can reach up to 80% in carefully chosen patients, depending on several factors, including the type of surgery (eg, hemispherectomy vs lesion- or lobectomy vs corpus callosotomy) and the underlying diagnosis.

Table 10-1

Common Etiologies of Refractory Epilepsy in Children

Structural	• Focal cortical dysplasia (including schizencephaly) • Congenital microcephaly and megalencephaly • Abnormal neuronal migration (including lissencephaly, heterotopia) • Sturge-Weber
Metabolic	• Disorders of neurotransmission (eg, pyridoxine dependent seizures, glucose transporter deficiency) • Disorders of energy metabolism (eg, mitochondrial disorders, disorders of pyruvate metabolism) • Storage disorders (including lysosomal disorders, peroxisomal disorders) • Disorders of amino acid and protein metabolism (eg, urea cycle disorders, amino and organic acidurias)
Other genetic	• Tuberous sclerosis complex • Angelman syndrome • Trisomies (21, 13) • *SCN1A* mutations (Dravet syndrome, GEFS +) • Progressive myoclonic epilepsies (including Lafora body disorder, Unverricht-Lundborg disease, DRPLA)
Inflammatory/ Autoimmune	• Rasmussen's encephalitis • Multisystemic autoimmune/connective tissue disorders (including systemic lupus erythematosus)
Other acquired	• Hypoxic ischemic encephalopathy • Trauma • Stroke • Tumor • Mesial temporal sclerosis

SCN1A: neuronal voltage-gated sodium channel alpha subunit type 1; GEFS+: generalized epilepsy with febrile seizure plus; DRPLA: dentatorubral-pallidoluysian atrophy.

Reprinted from *Semin Pediatr Neurol,* 18(3), Skjei KL, Dlugos DJ, The evaluation of treatment resistant epilepsy, 150-170, Copyright 2011, with permission from Elsevier.

Table 10-2

Three-Tier Laboratory Evaluation for Treatment-Resistant Epilepsy Secondary to Suspected Metabolic Disorder

	Tier 1	*Tier 2*	*Tier 3*
Blood	Acid base status (blood gas, anion gap) Ammonia Blood counts Creatine kinase Electrolytes (including calcium, magnesium) Glucose Lactate and pyruvate (arterial preferred) Liver function tests (including albumin and coagulation studies) Uric acid	Acylcarnitine profile (blood or plasma) Amino acids, quantitative (including homocysteine) Biotinidase Carnitine (free and total) TSH, free T4 VLCFA WBC lysosomal enzymes	Glycosylation studies Copper, ceruloplasmin Creatine and metabolites
Urine	Routine urinalysis (including ketones and reducing substances)	Acylglycines Amino acids Mucopolysaccharides Oligosaccharides Organic acids Sialic acid Sulphite test (bedside)	Creatine and metabolites Purine and pyrimidine panel (including uracil, hypoxanthine, and xanthine) Succinyladenosine SAICA riboside
CSF		Protein Glucose Cell count Lactate/pyruvate (quantitative) Quantitative amino acids (obtain together with plasma amino acids for comparison) Neurotransmitters	

(continued)

Table 10-2 (continued)

Three-Tier Laboratory Evaluation for Treatment-Resistant Epilepsy Secondary to Suspected Metabolic Disorder

	Tier 1	*Tier 2*	*Tier 3*
Other		Ophthalmic examination (vision, cherry red, optic atrophy, conjunct biopsy) Auditory exam	Skin biopsy Muscle biopsy

TSH: thyroid-stimulating hormone; VLCFA: very long chain fatty acid; WBC: white blood cells; SAICA: succinylaminoimidazolecarboxamide; CSF: cerebrospinal fluid.

Reprinted from *Semin Pediatr Neurol*, 18(3), Skjei KL, Dlugos DJ, The evaluation of treatment resistant epilepsy, 150-170, Copyright 2011, with permission from Elsevier.

Factors that make a patient a potentially good candidate for epilepsy surgery include the following:

- A single seizure type with:
  - Clear focal onset on EEG
  - An identifiable lesion on MRI (not involving eloquent cortex)
  - Concordance between imaging, EEG, neuropsychometric studies, and clinical (semiological) features

Presurgical evaluations must be thorough. Most include structural neuroimaging (such as MRI), LTM, neuropsychometric testing, functional imaging, and potentially intracranial EEG. MRIs should be performed with an established epilepsy protocol at a tertiary epilepsy center, as specific MRI sequences and slice-thickness may vary widely at outside institutions. If an MRI with epilepsy protocol has already been obtained and was negative, consider repeating it if significant time has passed, as changes in myelination and brain maturation may reveal a lesion that was previously hidden. Furthermore, some progressive disorders such as Rasmussen's encephalitis may initially be associated with a normal MRI.

Approximately 20% to 30% of patients with treatment-resistant partial epilepsy do not demonstrate abnormalities on conventional MRI. In the past, these patients were considered to be "nonlesional." However, more recent imaging techniques such as magnetoelectroencephalography (MEG), diffusion tensor imaging (DTI), and functional neuroimaging techniques (such as positron-emission tomography [PET], functional MRI, and single photon emission computed tomography [SPECT]) have begun to demonstrate areas of subtle abnormalities that are not picked up on routine MRI investigations. Such lesions may be amenable to surgical resection. In some instances, intracranial EEG may be needed to localize ictal onset.

If surgical intervention is not a possibility, the next question is, "Would a vagal nerve stimulator (VNS) or the ketogenic diet be a good alternative?" VNSs are subcutaneous programmable pacemakers that send mild, intermittent electrical impulses to the brain via the vagus nerve. They were approved by the Food and Drug Administration (FDA) in 1997 as adjunctive therapy for refractory partial onset seizures in adults and adolescents over 12 years of age. More than 65,000 patients worldwide have been implanted with VNSs. Although expensive, this treatment is approved by insurance companies because of a decrease in emergency department (ED) visits and hospitalizations. Surgical placement of the device can be performed either as an inpatient or outpatient procedure. The most common side effects are alterations in voice (hoarseness, deepening or quivering of voice), throat pain (during stimulation), cough, shortness of breath, gastroesophageal reflux, and sleep apnea. Most side effects occur only during stimulation, generally diminish over time, and/or may be decreased or eliminated by the adjustment of VNS parameter settings. More serious side effects that have been reported include vocal cord paralysis, aspiration pneumonia, and cardiac arrhythmias.

Current studies examining vagal nerve stimulation in children less than 12 years of age (an off-label use) demonstrate a > 50% seizure reduction in about 55% of children with partial or generalized epilepsy, and the benefits of vagal nerve stimulation appear to increase over time.[4] Although vagal nerve stimulation appears to be more effective in refractory partial epilepsy, they can also significantly decrease seizure frequency in patients with generalized epilepsies. Although some studies show that a small percentage of patients may become seizure free with a VNS, it is generally considered a palliative procedure. It is important to counsel families that some patients show no significant improvement in seizure frequency. Of note, VNS therapy does not affect AED requirements and has no effect on mortality (including sudden unexpected death in epilepsy).

The ketogenic diet is another intervention beyond AEDs and surgery that is used to control refractory epilepsy. It is a diet high in fat, low in carbohydrates, and providing adequate protein needed to sustain growth. The ratio in grams of fat to grams of protein and carbohydrates combined typically ranges between 3:1 and 4:1, and must be adhered to strictly. The ketogenic diet has been shown to be effective in controlling seizures both in focal and generalized epilepsies, with 40% to 50% of patients showing a greater than 50% reduction in seizure frequency, and 10% to 30% or more with a greater than 90% reduction in seizure burden. The ketogenic diet has also been shown to have a positive impact on alertness and cognition in many children with epilepsy. The ketogenic diet can be particularly helpful for epileptic encephalopathies such as migrating partial epilepsy of infancy, Lennox-Gastaut syndrome, and severe myoclonic epilepsy of infancy (Dravet syndrome). It should be considered early in myoclonic-astatic epilepsy (Doose syndrome) and is the first-line treatment in particular metabolic disorders, including glucose transporter type 1 deficiency and pyruvate dehydrogenase deficiency. It is contraindicated in patients with disorders of fatty acid oxidation and carnitine metabolism, which must be ruled out prior to diet initiation.

In addition to the above therapeutic options, continued drug trials remain a viable option in the management of children with refractory epilepsy. Dozens of AEDs with widely varying mechanisms of action are currently available, with new medications appearing all the time. Indeed, over the past 5 years, 6 new medications have been approved by the FDA for the treatment of epilepsy. The majority of these have novel mechanisms of action, allowing for fresh approaches and rational polypharmacy in even the most intractable cases.

Summary

When presented with refractory epilepsy, I ask myself the following questions: (1) Is it truly epilepsy? (2) Is it truly refractory? (3) Is there an underlying metabolic and/or genetic disorder that might suggest or preclude certain treatment options? (4) Is the patient potentially a surgical candidate? If the answer to question 4 is no, or if the patient remains refractory following epilepsy surgery, then (5) Would VNS or the ketogenic diet be helpful? And finally, (6) What novel medications have not been tried? Management of refractory epilepsy is, by definition, challenging. But with each passing year, more therapeutic options avail themselves, and the outlook is only as bleak as it is perceived to be by the practitioner.

References

1. Arts WF, Brouwer OF, Peters AC, et al. Course and prognosis of childhood epilepsy: 5-year follow-up of the Dutch study of epilepsy in childhood. *Brain.* 2004;127:1774-1784.
2. Skjei KL, Dlugos DJ. The evaluation of treatment resistant epilepsy. *Semin Pediatr Neurol.* 2011;18(3):150-170.
3. Skjei K, Harding B, Holland K, Clancy R, Porter B, Marsh E. Mild malformations of cortical development in patients with *SCN1A* mutations. Submitted for publication.
4. Morris GL 3rd, Gloss D, Buchhalter J, Mack KJ, Nickels K, Harden C. Evidence-based guideline update: vagus nerve stimulation for the treatment of epilepsy: report of the Guideline Development Subcommittee of the American Academy of Neurology. *Neurology.* 2013;81(16):1453-1459. doi: 10.1212/WNL.0b013e3182a393d1.

CAN A CHILD WITH SEIZURES RECEIVE ALL VACCINATIONS?

Kashif Ali Mir, MD and Karen L. Skjei, MD

Vaccines decrease the burden of infectious disease and have dramatically reduced pediatric morbidity and mortality worldwide. Vaccines protect the children who receive them and those with whom they are in contact. They are licensed only after rigorous testing and, once in use, the US Centers for Disease Control (CDC) and US Food and Drug Administration continuously monitor their safety and efficacy.[1] It is recommended that healthy children receive all scheduled vaccinations.

Vaccines are not completely benign, however. Certain neurologic and non-neurologic conditions are seen with slightly higher incidence following administration of particular vaccines, including brachial neuritis and Guillain-Barré syndrome, although these complications are very rare. In addition, certain vaccines are also avoided in particular patient populations, such as those with immune deficiencies.

Of all recommended vaccines for children, there are only a few whose safety can be questioned in certain subpopulations of children with seizures. One such population is children with a history of prolonged, refractory febrile seizures. Febrile seizures usually occur between 3 months and 5 years of age. They are associated with fever, but without evidence of intracranial infection. Approximately 1 in 25 children will have at least one febrile seizure, and while the risk of developing epilepsy is low, the risk of a recurrent febrile seizure after the initial event is about 30% to 40%.

Two vaccines commonly associated with post-vaccination fevers have also been associated with an increased incidence of febrile seizures. One is the measles-mumps-rubella (MMR) vaccine. The MMR induces fever and febrile seizures 8 to 14 days after immunization (relative risk, 2.8; 95% confidence interval, 1.4 to 5.6).[2] This risk is even higher following vaccination with MMR plus varicella (MMRV). The CDC's Vaccine Safety Datalink study found that 7 to 10 days after the first dose of vaccination, the rate of febrile seizures was about 2 times higher among children who received MMRV vaccine than among children who received the MMR and varicella vaccines

Licht DJ, Ryan NR, eds. *Curbside Consultation in Pediatric Neurology: 49 Clinical Questions* (pp 51-53).

separately at the same visit. The Advisory Committee on Immunization Practices recommends children with a personal or family history of seizures of any etiology should be vaccinated with the MMR vaccine and the varicella vaccine separately.[1]

The second vaccine associated with an increased risk of febrile seizures is the diphtheria-pertussis-tetanus vaccine (DPT), which has been associated with an increased risk of febrile seizures on the day of vaccination (adjusted relative risk, 5.7; 95% confidence interval, 2.0 to 16.4). It was determined that the cellular pertussis component of the DPT vaccine was responsible for the increased risk of febrile seizures. The incidence of febrile seizures and status epilepticus (as well as other neurologic complications) decreased significantly following the transition to an acellular pertussis vaccination (DTaP) in 1991.[3] Although there remains an increased risk of febrile seizures with the first 2 DTaP-inactivated polio virus-*Haemophilus influenzae* type b vaccinations (given at 3 and 5 months of age), the absolute risk is small (< 4 per 100,000 vaccinations).

Children with severe myoclonic epilepsy of infancy (Dravet syndrome) are also at risk for seizure exacerbation following vaccinations. One of the hallmark characteristics of Dravet syndrome is its presentation in the first year of life with febrile seizures, often febrile status epilepticus. Even beyond infancy the seizures tend to remain exquisitely sensitive to elevations in temperature. Up to one-third of all patients with Dravet syndrome experience vaccination-related seizures, in particular, within the first 72 hours after DPT vaccinations. Interestingly, these seizures are not always associated with fever.

The CDC recommends that any child who experiences long or multiple seizures within 7 days after a dose of DPT or DTaP should not be given that vaccine again in the future, unless a cause other than the vaccine was found. Such individuals may still receive tetanus-diphtheria without pertussis (TD).[1] The CDC also recommends that vaccination with DTaP be delayed in any child with a known or suspected neurologic condition until that condition has been evaluated, treatment initiated, and the condition stabilized. This includes children with an evolving seizure disorder (eg, uncontrolled epilepsy and infantile spasms) or a history of seizures that has not been evaluated. A family history of seizures or other neurologic diseases, or stable or resolved neurologic conditions (eg, controlled idiopathic epilepsy), are not contraindications to vaccination.

All parents should be counseled about the possibility of fever after receiving certain vaccines and educated on timing and measures to control it. Many practitioners suggest using acetaminophen at the time of vaccination, primarily to reduce the minor systemic effects of the vaccine. Given the increased risk of febrile seizures following certain vaccines, it would seem plausible that the use of antipyretics might decrease the incidence of febrile seizures following vaccination. However, there are no randomized clinical trials or observational studies to support this practice.[4]

Thus, with few exceptions, the answer to the question, "Can a child with seizures receive all scheduled vaccinations?" is "yes." Vaccinations are not contraindicated in the vast majority of children with a history of seizures or epilepsy. Furthermore, they are not necessarily contraindicated in patients with a history of seizures after immunizations. However, we agree with the CDC's recommendation that any child with a history of prolonged seizures or status epilepticus following a previous immunization should not be given that vaccine in the future. Similarly, patients with Dravet syndrome or a history of prolonged, refractory febrile seizures may be advised to avoid vaccination with DPT and MMR/MMRV. Finally, children with an uncontrolled or evolving seizure disorder or one that has not yet been evaluated should not receive the cellular or acellular pertussis vaccine, although they may still receive TD.[1]

References

1. Centers for Disease Control and Prevention. Vaccines & immunizations. Available at: http://www.cdc.gov/vaccines/. Accessed August 14, 2014.
2. Barlow WE, Davis RL, Glasser JW, et al. The risk of seizures after receipt of whole-cell pertussis or measles, mumps, and rubella vaccine. *N Engl J Med.* 2001;345(9):656-661.
3. Kuno-Sakai H, Kimura M. Safety and efficacy of acellular pertussis vaccine in Japan, evaluated by 23 years of its use for routine immunization. *Pediatr Int.* 2004;46(6):650-655.
4. Davis RL, Barlow W. Placing the risk of seizures with pediatric vaccines in a clinical context. *Paediatr Drugs.* 2003;5(11):717-722.

What Do I Do When a Child Seizes in My Office? Can a Child Die From Seizures?

Mai T. Dang, MD, PhD and Ernest Barbosa, MD

In a private pediatric practice, approximately one-quarter of patients you will see will have some neurologic issue. As many as 150,000 children and adolescents in the United States will seek medical attention each year for evaluation of a newly occurring seizure. In addition, approximately 4% of all children in the United States experience at least one convulsive episode associated with a febrile illness before the age of 5 years.[1] Thus, it would not be surprising to see a child have a seizure in your office. Fortunately, most seizures are brief and not life threatening, typically lasting 1 to 2 minutes. When a child has a seizure in your office, remain calm because you are the one expected to be in charge. Move the child to a safe area where he or she cannot be harmed while seizing. Lay the child on one side and slightly leaning forward so that saliva and vomit can come out of the mouth and not obstruct the airway. Do not place anything in the child's mouth. If you do, you run the risk of breaking teeth, causing vomiting, or being bitten. If you suspect airway obstruction from a foreign body, sweep the mouth with one finger to pull out the object. A seizing child cannot swallow his or her tongue.

Do not panic if you see perioral cyanosis. Remember that the brain cannot seize without adequate oxygen. The cyanosis is typically attributed to seizure-induced autonomic dysregulation causing peripheral vascular constriction. A seizing child may also have brief episodes of shallow breathing or brief periods of breathing cessation during the event that typically self-resolves. You do not need to give oxygen in the office for seizures. When the seizure stops, the child's breathing pattern will normalize. In an otherwise normal child in your office, there is virtually no risk for death during the seizure. Besides the drowning risk if a child has a seizure while in a body of water, mortality in children from epilepsy is extremely low. Analyses of deaths associated with seizures show that children most at risk for sudden unexplained death in epilepsy (SUDEP) are those with symptomatic epilepsy (ie, caused by widespread brain damage), refractory generalized

Licht DJ, Ryan NR, eds. *Curbside Consultation in Pediatric Neurology: 49 Clinical Questions* (pp 55-56).
© 2016 Taylor & Francis Group.

tonic-clonic epilepsy, and those who have failed surgical intervention for their epilepsy.[2,3] We generally talk about SUDEP only with families whose children are in the high-risk group.

When the seizing child in your office is in a safe place and positioned properly, you should check the time while you are observing and waiting for the seizure to end. If the seizure should last for 5 minutes or more, you can administer Diastat (diazepam) rectally, which can be dosed according to the manufacturer's suggestion. Five minutes is not a magic number, but over the years, clinicians have noted that the longer a seizure lasts, the more difficult it is to stop. A patient with a first-time seizure will need to be treated differently from a patient with known epilepsy. Patients who have known epilepsy and are having a typical seizure with a predictable course can be monitored in the office until they return to baseline. At any point that you are uncomfortable with caring for this child, emergency medical services (EMS) should be called and the child should be evaluated in the emergency department (ED). The child with a first-time seizure should be evaluated in the ED and will also need to be observed there until he or she returns to baseline. The most important 3 pieces of information to relay to EMS and the ED are the following:

1. Identify the patient either as a known epilepsy patient or one who does not have a diagnosis of epilepsy. If the patient has known epilepsy, let the new care team know which medications and doses he or she is taking.

2. Identify the type of seizure: either provoked or unprovoked. Examples of provoking factors include infection with fever (ie, infection in the throat, ears, lungs, and vomiting and diarrhea) and hypo- or hyperglycemia.

3. Describe the seizure. Did the seizure start focally with eye or head deviation to one side or shaking of one side of the body? Focal seizures can very rapidly generalize, but how the seizure starts will be important for medication selection.

Finally, reassure the family that a brief seizure does not cause brain damage. One must seize for hours before changes can occur in the brain that cause clinical symptoms. Parents can be directed to the Epilepsy Foundation website at www.epilepsyfoundation.org for more information on seizures.

References

1. Hauser WA. The prevalence and incidence of convulsive disorders in children. *Epilepsia.* 1994;35(Suppl 2):S1-S6.
2. Sillanpaa M, Shinnar S. Long-term mortality in childhood-onset epilepsy. *N Engl J Med.* 2010;363(26):2522-2529.
3. Langan Y, Nashef L, Sander JW. Case-control study of SUDEP. *Neurology.* 2005;64(7):1131-1133.

SECTION II

ALTERED MENTAL STATUS

METABOLIC, INFECTIOUS, TOXINS/DRUGS/CONCUSSION

What Is a Breath-Holding Spell? Can It Be Treated?

Donna J. Stephenson, MD

Breath-holding spells (BHS) result in temporary loss of consciousness with or without convulsion that is terrifying for parents to witness. Consultation with a pediatrician is often solicited. Parental anxiety is often very high; parents become worried that the spells could lead to the death of their child. A pediatrician's role is to establish the correct diagnosis with confidence, convey the diagnosis and natural history and outcome, treat if necessary, and, most important, provide reassurance to worried families.

BHS are typically seen between 1 and 3 years of age. Onset for cyanotic spells is usually between 6 and 12 months of age. If onset is after age 2, other diagnoses may need to be considered. Males are affected as often as females. There is another family member with BHS in 20% to 35% of patients. The frequency of spells ranges from a few per year to more than daily spells. Increased frequency of spells is more common in males, and males tend to have more spells earlier than females.[1]

BHS have historically been differentiated into "cyanotic" and "pallid" types. Cyanotic spells predominate; pallid spells are seen less often. Both cyanotic and pallid spells can occur in the same individual, and at times the differentiation of the 2 types is unclear, leading to a designation of a "mixed" type spell. In a cyanotic BHS the child first becomes angry, upset, or frustrated. Crying occurs with an excessive expiratory effort. At the end of a long expiration respiratory effort appears to cease. The child stills, becomes progressively more red or blue (mostly perioral), and is unresponsive. Often there is generalized stiffening, with or without arching of the back, eyes rolling back in the head, and/or generalized tonic jerking of the extremities. The convulsions associated with BHS are usually brief, lasting less than 30 seconds after which the child relaxes and begins to breathe normally. Color returns to normal within a few minutes. The child will wake easily and seem normally reactive but may go to sleep after a more severe spell. In pallid spells there is often an antecedent mild injury (bump to a part of the body, often the head) or emotional shock. The

Licht DJ, Ryan NR, eds. *Curbside Consultation in Pediatric Neurology: 49 Clinical Questions* (pp 59-61).

Table 13-1
Characteristics of Breath-Holding Spells and Seizures

	Breath-Holding Spells	Seizure
Precipitating factor	Usually present	Unusual
Respiratory effort	Absent	Present
Convulsion	Possible, short	1 to 2 minutes
Post-ictal state	Brief (seconds)	Prolonged (minutes)

child immediately becomes pale or mildly cyanotic, becomes limp, and collapses. Breathing may be very shallow or not detectable. Pallid spells may also result in stiffening or convulsive movements of brief duration. The spells end with a fairly rapid (seconds) return to normal responsiveness, although the child may want to sleep.

Both types of BHS are thought to represent a mild dysregulation of the autonomic nervous system. The pathophysiology of the cyanotic type is best conceptualized as respiratory inhibition with little cardiac inhibition (largely sympathetically mediated) and for the pallid type a major cardiac inhibition (asystole) with little respiratory inhibition (parasympathetically driven). These conceptualizations are supported by several studies suggesting children with pallid BHS have lower resting heart rates and a greater likelihood of asystole with ocular compression testing (which causes a brainstem-mediated reflex arc and increases vagal tone).

Obtaining a very detailed history of the spells is crucial in establishing the diagnosis. Gathering the history firsthand from those who witnessed the spell(s) will provide the most accurate information. This may mean contacting care providers other than the parents. The goal of the history is to develop a sequential playback of events. The setting in which the attack occurs, the activity level/state of the child, and the presence or absence of a precipitating event or injury may all help determine whether the spell was triggered or spontaneous. The initial physical signs of a spell should be sought out as they are the best clues to etiologic diagnosis. Having the parent/witness act out the spell may elicit a previously unrecognized detail. Observations such as whether eyes were open or closed, rolled back, or deviated are important. Breathing, coloring, and pulse rate if available are also important. Response level, stiffening or limpness, and focal or generalized shaking may point the clinician in a diagnostic direction. Document the interval from the spell end to normal responsiveness. In most BHS the child becomes responsive and aware within about 30 seconds, which may help differentiate BHS from seizures after which post-ictal recovery is often minutes at a minimum. Do not forget to ask about family history including not only BHS but seizures, cardiac arrhythmias, and sudden death.

The examination of children with BHS is normal, although if you are lucky you might trigger a spell just by pulling out a stethoscope.

It is imperative for BHS to be differentiated from seizure (Table 13-1). A thorough history will usually point the provider in the right diagnostic direction. In seizures stiffening of all or part of the body followed by convulsive movements will precede the cyanosis. The convulsive movements in seizure generally last in the range of minutes, not seconds. A post-ictal state is often longer than 30 seconds. Seizures are in general not provoked by mild trauma or emotion. More serious cardiac disease such as congenital heart disease may be associated with alteration of consciousness but should have symptoms provoked by exercise or physical findings suggestive of structural abnormality. The possibility of prolonged QT syndrome may be suggested by family history or no clear-cut antecedent event before each spell.

Ancillary testing is usually unnecessary to establish the diagnosis. In BHS, the history is sufficient for the diagnosis in the majority of cases. If there is a suspicion of epileptic seizure, an electroencephalogram (EEG) can be obtained. A standard EEG has the advantage of being readily available in most communities and being tolerated well by the child. However, there are several confounders with almost any EEG result. If the EEG is normal it neither confirms nor refutes the diagnosis of either epilepsy or BHS. If the EEG is abnormal it does suggest an increased likelihood of seizure but unless a spell is captured on the EEG a diagnosis of epilepsy cannot be truly confirmed. If the spells are quite frequent, a 24-hour video-correlated EEG may be definitive.

Ocular compression has historically been used during a standard EEG to evaluate for cardiac (vagal) reactivity via the trigeminal reflex arc. This has been studied in small patient series and found to have high specificity but low sensitivity. It is currently not recommended as part of an evaluation for BHS.

It is recognized that iron deficiency anemia is common in children with BHS. It is theorized that anemia may worsen autonomic control mechanisms. Treatment of iron deficiency is recommended for severe BHS at a daily dose of 6 mg/kg. Two of 3 studies showed statistically significant improvement in BHS over a minimum of 3 months. Side effects of iron supplementation are few but include nausea, vomiting, diarrhea, and change in stool color.

Many medications have been tried for severe BHS, including many antiepileptic drugs. There are no Food and Drug Administration-approved medications for the treatment of BHS. Studies are few; no medication has been deemed effective in the reduction of BHS spells. A recent open-label study of piracetam (not available in the United States at present) suggested effectiveness without significant side effects.

BHS are a developmental phenomenon. Most BHS resolve between 3 and 4 years of age. It is unusual for spells to last past 7 years of age. There is some suggestion that children with BHS are at slightly increased risk of developing syncope later in life.

Reference

1. DiMario FJ Jr. Prospective study of children with cyanotic and pallid breath-holding spells. *Pediatrics.* 2001;107(2):265-269.

Suggested Readings

Azam M, Bhatti N, Shahab N. Piracetam in severe breath holding spells. *Int J Psychiatr Med.* 2008;38(2):195-201.

DiMario FJ Jr, Chee CM, Berman PH. Pallid breath-holding spells: evaluation of the autonomic nervous system. *Clin Pediatr (Phila).* 1990;29(1):17-24.

Mocan H, Yildiran A, Orhan F, Erduran E. Breath holding spells in 91 children and response to treatment with iron. *Arch Dis Child.* 1991;81(3):261-262.

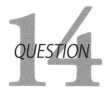

A MOTHER CALLS BECAUSE HER CHILD HAS HAD EPISODES OF CONFUSION OVER THE LAST WEEK BUT IS OTHERWISE ACTING NORMALLY. HOW SHOULD THE CHILD BE EVALUATED?

Caitlin Rollins, MD

Confusion is an imprecise term that may refer to a wide range of symptoms including altered consciousness, unusual behaviors, or focal neurological deficits such as language disturbance. Start by asking an open-ended yet specific question to characterize the child's symptoms: "Can you tell me what happened during the most recent episodes?" If the parent did not witness the episodes, speak directly with an observer. Even better, if episodes are frequent, ask the family to videotape them. Many different entities can present as episodic confusion, and a good description is often the best diagnostic tool.

Once you clarify the nature of the confusion, use additional details to narrow your differential (Table 14-1). First, consider the patient's age. Some diagnoses are more common in specific age groups (eg, toxic ingestions usually occur in young children). Second, ask if the child or a family member ever experienced a similar episode. These details may be omitted amid an acute concern. Next, identify the setting where they occur. Agitation early in the night suggests sleep terrors while movements provoked by sleep deprivation may be seizures. Finally, assess risk factors for neurological disease such as prematurity, head trauma, or infection. You may be surprised how well you can narrow the differential during the initial phone call.

After obtaining a thorough history, consider specific diagnoses. Seizures can cause paroxysmal confusion, either during the seizure itself or in the post-ictal phase. Parents may describe staring, behavioral arrest, lip smacking, or drooling. Spells are often stereotyped with a similar pattern each time. Determine duration and frequency. Ask about extremity or mouth movements suggesting automatisms (stereotyped, nonpurposeful movements), gaze deviation, head version, and incontinence. Consider the time of day—do episodes happen at night, upon awakening, while asleep? Family history may be positive in syndromes like absence or juvenile myoclonic epilepsy (JME). Try to classify the seizure type. While typical absence seizures involve staring or blinking

Licht DJ, Ryan NR, eds. *Curbside Consultation in Pediatric Neurology: 49 Clinical Questions* (pp 63-67). © 2016 Taylor & Francis Group.

Table 14-1
Five Key Questions

1. Could you describe the most recent episodes?
2. How old is the child (might he or she have taken something—what medications are in the house)?
3. Has anyone in the family ever experienced anything similar?
4. What is the setting where the spells occur most often (eg, during sleep, transitions, while awake)?
5. Are there any risk factors such as prematurity, head injury, or recent infection?

for a few seconds repeatedly throughout the day without prodrome or post-ictal phase, absence status epilepticus lasts longer and can present as confusion. Ask about prior staring or blinking suggesting undiagnosed seizures. Inquire whether the child pauses while speaking or only when passively listening. With daydreaming the child may stare but would not typically do so mid-sentence. If the parent describes post-ictal confusion, consider atypical absence seizures or focal dyscognitive seizures. Dyscognitive seizures are those that affect consciousness or awareness (focal dyscognitive roughly corresponds to complex partial from the prior epilepsy classification). Compared to absence seizures, focal dyscognitive seizures usually last minutes rather than seconds, are accompanied by automatisms or abnormal movements, and have an aura or post-ictal phase. Patients may lack recall for blocks of time or notice an injury without a known mechanism. Finally, consider other common seizure syndromes. JME typically begins as morning muscle jerks (eg, dropping items while preparing for school). Myoclonus may go unrecognized but alcohol or sleep deprivation can trigger a generalized seizure with confusion observed post-ictally. Similarly, confusion associated with nocturnal arousals or awakening could represent nocturnal frontal lobe seizures or the post-ictal phase of secondarily generalized seizures in benign epilepsy with centrotemporal spikes.

When evaluating nocturnal confusion, consider parasomnias. Parasomnias arise out of rapid eye movement (REM) or non-REM (NREM) sleep. In children, NREM-associated parasomnias such as confusional arousals, sleep terrors, and sleepwalking are most likely to present as confusion. With confusional arousals, the child sits up, appears disoriented, then returns to sleep. Sleep terrors are similar but accompanied by autonomic symptoms like fear, flushing, tachycardia, or motor behavior. In contrast to nightmares, children are generally inconsolable and do not recall the episode. Sleepwalking manifests as crawling or walking in an altered state of arousal sometimes with unusual behaviors. NREM parasomnias typically occur during the first third of the night, while REM-associated phenomena such as nightmares are more likely during the latter half. Confusional arousals and sleep terrors occur in younger children, age 4 to 7 years, while sleepwalking peaks around age 8 to 12 years. If you suspect parasomnia, also consider seizures. Although nocturnal frontal lobe seizures can be similar to parasomnias with bizarre behavior, complex movements, or vocalizations, generally seizures are more frequent, stereotyped, and randomly distributed through the night than parasomnias. Both may be inherited. Unlike epilepsy, childhood parasomnias rarely require treatment. Instead, minimize triggers such as sleep deprivation or breathing disorders and reassure parents to simply ensure the child's safety during episodes.

Migraine is another common pediatric diagnosis that can manifest with confusion. Migraines typically last longer than seizures, are usually (though not always) associated with headache, and may include nausea, vomiting, photophobia, or phonophobia. Family history is often present. Migraine aura symptoms that may be perceived as confusion include visual hallucinations, dysphasia, or reduced alertness. Also consider variants like confusional migraine, hemiplegic migraine, and basilar-type migraine (see Question 21). Particularly in children who cannot articulate their experiences, these symptoms may manifest as confusion.

While focal neurological deficits can occur with migraines, they raise concern for a vascular event such as transient ischemic attack (TIA) or stroke. A history of cardiac, hematologic, or rheumatologic disease or recent head/neck trauma increases suspicion for a vascular etiology. If the mother describes preserved alertness with language disturbance (eg, not understanding spoken language), consider aphasia. When a nearly occluded vessel causes intermittent ischemia, a child may experience stereotyped spells, not unlike seizures. With embolic events, symptoms usually differ with each episode. Inquire about other focal neurological symptoms such as altered gait, reduced extremity use, or discoordination. Parents may not associate the other focal symptoms with the confusion and thus may not describe them unless asked. Distinguishing TIA from seizure or migraine can be challenging. Usually seizures have positive phenomena while migraine or TIA involve a deficit. If the deficit lasts hours with the patient returning to baseline each time, migraine is more likely. On the other hand, brief, repeated spells of variable semiology lasting minutes suggest emboli. Stereotyped spells suggest a single seizure focus, stenotic vessel causing recurrent ischemia, or migraine.

Finally, always consider toxic ingestion. Accidental toxic ingestions are most common in mobile children under 4 years and those with prior ingestions. In older children consider intentional ingestion (eg, substance abuse or overdose). Rarely parents may surreptitiously administer substances as in Munchausen syndrome by proxy. Ask about medications and chemicals available in the home. Benzodiazepines, antiepileptic drugs, and antidepressants may impair consciousness. Amphetamines or cocaine could produce agitation. Hypoglycemic agents may reduce alertness or provoke seizures. Accompanying features such as changes in respiration, pupil size, skin turgor, or muscle tone may guide you to a specific agent or class.

The next step in your evaluation is triaging the acuity. If ischemia is possible, you must have the child evaluated emergently. While strokes and TIA are unusual, early treatment is critical. Prolonged episodes of altered consciousness suggesting seizure also merit emergent treatment. While status epilepticus is usually defined as at least 30 minutes, children with spells lasting 5 minutes or more are at high risk of evolving to status epilepticus. Other features prompting emergency referral include increasing frequency or duration of possible seizures, concern for toxic ingestion or metabolic deviation, or suspicion of serious infection.

If you rule out emergencies based on the history, you will next want to perform a complete examination. Search for any evidence of head injury. Abnormal vital signs, unusual odors, or altered pupil size may hint at toxic ingestion. Ensure there is no papilledema. Another key focus is to identify subtle evidence of a persistent neurological impairment. Findings such as field cut, mild weakness, or sensory changes may go unnoticed by family members. If you suspect absence seizures, try hyperventilating the child for 3 minutes using a pinwheel or a sheet of paper to trigger an episode. You'll still want to confirm the diagnosis with an electroencephalogram (EEG).

Target your workup based on history and examination. If there is concern for electrolyte abnormalities or infection, order a metabolic panel or complete blood count with differential. In many cases of metabolic derangement or systemic illness confusion would be persistent, not episodic. Have a low threshold for sending toxicology screens. If you suspect seizures, request a sleep-deprived EEG capturing wakefulness and sleep. For focal seizures, obtain brain magnetic resonance imaging (MRI) to determine whether seizures are symptomatic of underlying

Table 14-2
Selected Differential Diagnosis

- Seizure
  - Absence seizure
  - Absence status epilepticus
  - Focal dyscognitive seizure
  - Post-ictal state
  - Possibly secondary to underlying familial syndrome, structural abnormality, infection, mass
- Migraine
  - Confusional migraine
  - Hemiplegic migraine with aphasia
  - Basilar-type migraine
- Vascular
  - Transient ischemic attack
  - Stroke
  - May relate to cardiac, hematologic, or rheumatologic disease, moyamoya, traumatic dissection
- Toxic
  - Accidental ingestion
  - Substance abuse
  - Medication side effect
- Metabolic
  - Hypoglycemia
  - Inborn error of metabolism
- Sleep-related
  - Night terrors
  - Confusional arousals
- Psychological
  - Panic attacks
  - Psychosis
  - Nonepileptic paroxysmal events (eg, functional disorders)
- Immunologic
  - Acute disseminated encephalomyelitis
  - Multiple sclerosis
  - Paraneoplastic process
- Intussusception

pathology. Any persistent focal neurological deficit raises suspicion for a structural abnormality, and MRI is indicated. Finally, do not forget to keep a broad differential. Etiologies of confusion range from intussusception in an infant to psychiatric disorders in adolescence, and maintaining a broad scope will maximize the likelihood of correctly identifying the underlying cause (Table 14-2).

Suggested Readings

Berg AT, Berkovic SF, Brodie MJ, et al. Revised terminology and concepts for organization of seizures and epilepsies: report of the ILAE Commission on Classification and Terminology. *Epilepsia.* 2010;51(4):676-685.

Hirtz D, Ashwal S, Berg A, et al. Practice parameter: evaluating a first nonfebrile seizure in children: report of the quality standards subcommittee of the American Academy of Neurology, the Child Neurology Society, and the American Epilepsy Society. *Neurology.* 2000;55(5):616-623.

Roach ES, Golomb MR, Adams R, et al. Management of stroke in infants and children: a scientific statement from a special writing group of the American Heart Association Stroke Council and the Council on Cardiovascular Disease in the Young. *Stroke.* 2008;39(9):2644-2691.

Tinuper P, Bisulli F, Provini F. The parasomnias: mechanisms and treatment. *Epilepsia.* 2012;53(Suppl 7):12-19.

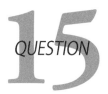

A CHILD HAS HAD A PROGRESSIVE DECLINE IN SCHOOL PERFORMANCE OVER THE LAST FEW MONTHS. HOW SHOULD THIS BE EVALUATED?

Xilma R. Ortiz-Gonzalez, MD, PhD

By far, the most common reasons for decline in school performance include anything from psychosocial stressors (divorce, death of a loved one or pet, new school, or bullying) to psychiatric disease (depression). These should be investigated first. But if the degree or rate of decline raises suspicion for cognitive deterioration, it is prudent to consider the possibility that a neurologic condition may be presenting insidiously. Particularly if the symptoms seem progressive or there is involvement of other organ systems, further evaluation is warranted. Visual abnormalities, cardiomyopathy, and liver involvement are among the symptoms commonly associated with some neurodegenerative disorders. Clinical course is important to consider, as a relapsing course will be more suggestive of an inflammatory/autoimmune etiology. A progressive course is more concerning for metabolic disorders, including leukodystrophies.

Initial evaluation should include neurological examination and neuroimaging (brain magnetic resonance imaging). Besides the cognitive involvement, it is important to identify whether other neurologic symptoms are present, such as seizures, movement disorders, eye movement abnormalities, or ataxia. Table 15-1 lists disorders to be considered in the differential diagnosis, along with distinguishing clinical or laboratory features. This list is most relevant for children and adolescents without a significant prior neurologic history. There are also several disorders that usually present before school age that are addressed in this chapter and addressed elsewhere,[1] such as metabolic disorders (ie, Tay-Sachs, Hurler's), severe epileptic encephalopathies that may have a regression component (Rett's syndrome), and more severe leukodystrophy syndromes (Pelizaeus-Merzbacher disease). If the child has a history of significant developmental delay, seizures, microcephaly, etc, the differential shall be expanded accordingly. Next are some clinical scenarios in which school decline may be among the presenting complaints to the pediatrician and that shall prompt further investigation.

Licht DJ, Ryan NR, eds. *Curbside Consultation in Pediatric Neurology: 49 Clinical Questions* (pp 69-74). © 2016 Taylor & Francis Group.

Table 15-1

Conditions That May Present With Neuropsychiatric Decline in Childhood or Adolescence

	Disorder	*Distinguishing Features*
Metabolic	Wilson's disease	Hepatopathy, Kayser-Fleischer rings, low serum ceruloplasmin, high urinary cooper, hemolytic anemia, movement disorder (ranging from tremors, choreo-athethosis, dystonia) Onset: mid-childhood to adulthood
	Lafora's disease	Generalized myoclonus and/or generalized tonic-clonic seizures, visual hallucinations (occipital seizures), photosensitivity in EEG, dysarthria, ataxia Onset: teenage years
	Mitochondrial disorders	± Lactic acidosis, decompensation/regression exacerbated by illness, MRI abnormalities, heterogenous with symptoms that may include GI dysmotility, hepatopathy, cardiomyopathy, sensorineural hearing loss, optic atrophy, ptosis, pigmentary retinopathy, ophthalmoplegia, stroke-like episodes, seizures, myopathy, exercise intolerance
	Niemann-Pick C	Vertical upgaze palsy, neonatal liver disease, progressive ataxia, dysarthria, dystonia, and seizures; biochemical profile[a] Onset: mid childhood to adulthood
	Neuroacanthocytosis	Acanthocytosis in RBC, compensated hemolysis, elevated CK, progressive chorea, psychiatric symptoms, cognitive decline, seizures, cardiomyopathy, arrhythmias, X-linked inheritance Onset: late childhood to adulthood
	Neuronal ceroid-lipofuscinoses)	Lysosomal disorder, visual loss (progressive retinopathy), seizures (particularly myoclonic), progressive dystonia, dysphagia; onset varies according to infantile, childhood, and juvenile forms Variants may present in adulthood or without visual loss

(continued)

Table 15-1 (continued)

Conditions That May Present With Neuropsychiatric Decline in Childhood or Adolescence

	Disorder	*Distinguishing Features*
	Neurodegeneration with brain iron accumulation	Group of diseases characterized by movement disorder (dystonia, chore-athetosis, rigidity), MRI shows focal iron accumulation in basal ganglia
Inflammatory/ autoimmune	Hashimoto's encephalopathy	Relapsing course (can be subacute or chronic), seizures, tremor, hallucinations, elevated anti-TPO and anti-TG titers, euthryroid or subclinical hypothyroidism, reported age of onset ranges from 8 to 86
	CNS vasculitis	Inflammatory markers, relapsing course, multifocal lesions on MRI, angiogram, biopsy
	Neuropsychiatric lupus	Arthritis, malar rash, glomerulonephritis, photosensitivity
		Variable CNS features may include: acute confusional state, transverse myelitis, seizures, headaches, cranial neuropathy, cerebral venous sinus thrombosis, white matter lesions
	Antiphospholipid antibodies syndrome	May be secondary in patients with SLE, but also occurs isolated (primary), movement disorder (chorea), thrombosis, TIA, seizures; serology[b]
	NMDA receptor encephalitis	Acute to subacute severe psychiatric presentation, orofacial dyskinesias, seizures, autonomic instability, anti-NMDA serology in CSF
Infectious/ post-infectious	HIV encephalopathy	HIV serology, opportunistic infections, CD4 counts
	Subacute sclerosing panencephalitis	Rapid decline, may present with vision complaints (necrotizing retinitis) and myoclonic jerks progressing over weeks to months to comatose state; periodic generalized complexes in EEG, history of measles[c]

(continued)

Table 15-1 (continued)

Conditions That May Present With Neuropsychiatric Decline in Childhood or Adolescence

	Disorder	*Distinguishing Features*
White matter disease	Multiple sclerosis	Multifocal white matter lesions disseminated in space and time, clinical history of relapsing episodes, history or exam findings suggestive of optic neuritis
	Neuromyelitis optica	Optic neuritis, longitudinally extensive transverse myelitis, Aquaporin-4 serology
	Adrenoleukodystrophy	Boys <10 years old (X-linked), symmetric, posterior predominant white matter abnormalities, abnormal VLCFA, adrenal insufficiency
	Metachromatic leukodystrophy (juvenile form)	Hypertonia/spasticity, leukodystrophy on MRI sparing U fibers, arylsulfatase A deficiency
	Krabbe's (juvenile form)	Hypertonia/spasticity, irritability, leukodystrophy on MRI, galactocerebroside deficiency
Others	Landau-Kleffner syndrome	Epileptic encephalopathy, classically affecting language due to electric status epilepticus of sleep, usually history of epilepsy

aFibroblasts cultured from skin biopsy show impaired cholesterol esterification and positive filipin staining.
bAnticardiolipin immunoglobulin (Ig)G or IgM, lupus anticoagulant anti-b2-glycoprotein1 IgG.
cRare in United States but still many cases reported in Turkey, Papua New Guinea, and India.

EEG: electroencephalogram; MRI: magnetic resonance imaging; GI: gastrointestinal; RBC: red blood cells; CK: creatine kinase; anti-TPO: antithyroid peroxidase; anti-TG: antithyroglobulin; CNS: central nervous system; SLE: systemic lupus erythematosus; TIA: transient ischemic attack; NMDA: N-methyl-D-aspartate; CSF: cerebrospinal fluid; HIV: human immunodeficiency virus; VLCFA: very long chain fatty acid.

Case 1

An 8-year-old boy presents to his pediatrician with progressive academic difficulties and behavioral changes. He has developed aggressive behaviors, inattentiveness, and decline in his ability to read. The family is also concerned about him being more clumsy and bumping into things, particularly at night.

This case is concerning for a neurodegenerative process that may be resulting in cognitive decline, vision loss, and ataxia, such as Batten's disease. Often nighttime vision changes precede other neurologic symptoms. Other visual complaints include photophobia and difficulty reading. Ophthalmologic examination may reveal visual field deficits, loss of color vision, and retinal abnormalities. Electroretinogram may detect rod/cone dystrophy prior to funduscopic changes and may be helpful for earlier diagnosis.[2] Neurologic examination may reveal ataxia and hyperreflexia and should prompt neuroimaging and lysosomal enzyme testing.

Case 2

A 13-year-old boy, previously an honor student and with no prior psychiatric history, has developed progressive academic difficulties. A year ago he developed involuntary movements that family described as tics and unusual obsessive behaviors. Now he has developed paranoid delusions and visual hallucinations. As the pediatrician you think this is unusual, older than typical onset of tics for Tourette's and younger than typical for first psychotic episode. On exam you find splenomegaly and limited upgaze.

This is a common presentation for Niemann-Pick C, in which psychiatric symptoms, decline in school performance, and vertical supranuclear gaze palsy may precede more severe manifestations like cataplexy, seizures, ataxia, and dysphagia.[3] Splenomealy is present in the majority of juvenile-onset cases. Diagnosis is traditionally made by biochemical testing of cholesterol transport in cultured fibroblasts obtained from a skin biopsy, although with high clinical suspicion some now proceed directly to genetic testing. This is an autosomal recessive disorder, and 95% of patients are found to have mutations in Niemann-Pick disease, type C1 (*NPC1*) or *NPC2*. Early diagnosis is helpful not only for counseling but because of the recent development of treatments (miglustat) that although not curative may stabilize neurologic decline, particularly in patients with late juvenile-onset of disease.[4]

Case 3

A 16-year-old girl presents to your office for concerns of depression. Her mother states that she has become withdrawn and doesn't talk as much as her usual self. Mom is also concerned about her worsening grades in school and her handwriting getting worse. At times family has complained of trouble understanding her speech. You've known this girl since she was a baby and agree that her affect is flat and withdrawn, but you also note she barely speaks and her speech seems dysarthric. On further questioning she admits that her hands have been "shaky" for the last 6 months and this has made tasks like handwriting and brushing her teeth harder. She tries to avoid handwriting and types as much as possible, and this has caused some trouble in school. She used to love math but is having a hard time now keeping up her grades. She is also embarrassed because her speech sounds funny so she likes to remain quiet. On examination you notice a tremor at rest in her hands and decide to check some labs and refer to neurology. While waiting for her specialist appointment, the comprehensive metabolic panel comes back with elevated liver enzymes and the complete blood count shows mild anemia. You send copper and ceruloplasmin levels and arrange for expedited neurologic and ophthalmologic evaluation.

Dysarthria and distal tremor can be among the first and more common signs of neurologic decline in patients with Wilson's disease. Ophthalmologic evaluation for cooper deposits in the limbic region of the cornea known as Kayser-Fleischer rings is crucial, as they are seen in essentially all patients with neurologic involvement and 50% of patients who are asymptomatic or with primarily hepatic involvement.[5] Neurologic examination may also reveal ataxia, and motor abnormalities that include dystonia, chorea, tremor, or parkinsonism. The classical finding is a proximal tremor known as a wing-beating tremor; nevertheless, a distal high-frequency tremor that may look similar to an essential tremor is more common. It is important to have a high level of suspicion in the primary care setting as this is a treatable disorder, and patients diagnosed early and treated appropriately can have good outcomes.

References

1. Fenichel GM. *Clinical Pediatric Neurology: A Signs and Symptoms Approach.* 5th ed. Philadelphia, PA: Elsevier Saunders; 2005:ix, 414.
2. Collins J, Holder GE, Herbert H, Adams GG. Batten disease: features to facilitate early diagnosis. *Br J Ophthalmol.* 2006;90(9):119-124.
3. Vanier MT. Niemann-Pick diseases. *Handb Clin Neurol.* 2013;113:1717-1721.
4. Héron B, Valayannopoulos V, Baruteau J, et al. Miglustat therapy in the French cohort of paediatric patients with Niemann-Pick disease type C. *Orphanet J Rare Dis.* 2012;7:36.
5. Lorincz MT. Recognition and treatment of neurologic Wilson's disease. *Semin Neurol.* 2012;32(5):538-543.

SECTION III

HEADACHE

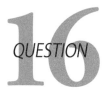

WHAT ARE THE MOST COMMON TYPES OF HEADACHES IN CHILDREN?

Christina Szperka, MD and Douglas Smith, MD

Headache is one of the most commonly encountered complaints in a pediatric neurology practice. Fundamentally, there are 2 different categories of headache: primary and secondary headaches. Secondary headaches are defined as those with an underlying direct etiology, including but not limited to infectious, traumatic, neoplastic, vascular, inflammatory, toxic, and metabolic causes. Primary headaches, by comparison, are defined by the absence of another etiology, and genetic factors are thought to play a role. Migraine and tension-type headaches are prototypical examples of primary headache disorders.

The foremost role of the clinician is to identify and treat causes of secondary headaches, the incidence of which varies considerably based on the age and location of presentation. Once secondary factors are excluded, the ability to treat a primary headache disorder appropriately depends on correct classification. Knowing the frequency, aggravating factors, and associated symptoms can lead to the correct diagnosis and ultimately, relief for the child.

How Often Do Headaches Occur in Children?

Headache is a nonspecific symptom that occurs in children with increasing frequency as they age. A survey of a general pediatric practice in the United Kingdom found that only 13.5% of 3-year-old children complained of having a headache within the past year; this number increases to 53.4% by 10 years of age.[1] This upward trend also appears with more bothersome headaches: a large study of American children found that 4.48% of children aged 4 to 5 years complained of frequent or severe headaches within the past year, increasing to 25% in the later teenage years, and shifts from being gender neutral to becoming female predominant post-puberty.[2]

Licht DJ, Ryan NR, eds. *Curbside Consultation in Pediatric Neurology: 49 Clinical Questions* (pp 77-80).
© 2016 Taylor & Francis Group.

The epidemiology of headache types depends on the setting of presentation. Children seen acutely by a primary care clinician or in the emergency department (ED) have a wide distribution of primary and secondary causes of headaches, whereas children seen in referral-based neurology or headache clinics are much more likely to have a primary headache disorder. A review summarizing multiple case series of children ages 2 to 18 presenting to the ED found that the majority of these children presented with secondary headaches, though many of the causes are relatively benign. Viral illness was the cause in 39% to 57%, 9% to 16% had sinusitis, 5.2% to 9% had viral meningitis, 4.9% to 9% had streptococcal pharyngitis, and 7.9% had post-concussive or post-traumatic headaches; only 16% to 18% were diagnosed with migraine.[3] Significant neurologic diseases such as neoplasm, hydrocephalus, shunt malfunction, and hemorrhage were uncommon, and nearly all of the patients with serious problems had either a history suggestive of significant pathology or an abnormal neurologic exam. A database study of children ages 5 to 17 presenting to the general practitioner in the United Kingdom with new-onset headache found similar results to the ED studies: A total of 19.2% were diagnosed with a primary headache disorder, and 1.1% had a serious secondary cause identified.[4] In contrast, the majority of patients presenting to pediatric neurology or a pediatric headache clinic are diagnosed with a primary headache disorder. A case series of 105 children under the age of 6 seen at an outpatient headache referral center in Italy reported that 70.4% were diagnosed with a primary headache disorder. In descending order the most frequent diagnoses were migraine, episodic tension-type headache, primary stabbing headache, and chronic daily headache.[5]

What Are the Signs and Symptoms of Secondary Headaches in Children?

Flags for secondary headache conditions in children can be summarized by the mnemonic "SNOOPY snoop4 secondary causes" (adapted from Dodick[6]):

- **S**ystemic disease signs or symptoms: Look for signs of infectious or inflammatory conditions, and consider substances including prescription medications.

- **N**eurologic disease signs or symptoms: Change in mental status, seizure, weakness, and gait abnormalities are concerning for serious central nervous system problems.[7] Vomiting, photophobia, phonophobia, and visual changes are nonspecific and can occur with many types of headaches. A full neurological examination, including funduscopic exam checking for papilledema, should be performed on all headache patients. When thinking about causes of increased intracranial pressure in children, remember that pseudotumor cerebri syndrome can cause increased pressure and papilledema without neoplasm.

- **O**nset sudden: "Thunderclap" onset, meaning headache that is maximal within seconds, is rare in children, but suggests bleeding, vascular causes, or intermittent obstruction of the flow of cerebrospinal fluid.

- **O**ccipital location: This can be concerning for posterior fossa tumor or Chiari malformation,[3] but occipital location of pain is also commonly seen in primary headaches.

- **P**attern:
  - Progressive or new: This is a risk factor for serious secondary causes, and imaging (preferably brain magnetic resonance imaging if safe) should be considered for any headache problem that started within the prior month, and for any headache problem that started in the prior 6 months where there is another flag for a secondary cause (lack of family history, abnormal exam, vomiting, etc).[7]

- ○ **P**arents: Lack of family history is a risk factor for secondary headache.[7] Most patients with migraine have a family history of migraine or other headaches, though it is sometimes necessary to ask specifically about menstrual and "sinus" headaches in order to learn about all family members with headache.

- ○ **P**recipitated by Valsalva: Many headaches are briefly worsened by bearing down, coughing, and sneezing. Headaches that are elicited only by these movements, or headaches that worsen significantly with these movements, may suggest a Chiari malformation or increased intracranial pressure.

- ○ **P**ositional: Pain worse when lying down, or pain that awakens the patient at night are concerning for increased intracranial pressure. Pain worse when upright suggests cerebrospinal fluid leak or orthostatic blood pressure problems. Pain worse with any activity, not specific to position, is consistent with migraine.

- • Years < 6: Young age is a risk factor for secondary headaches,[5] and it is difficult to obtain sufficient detail about the features of headache to make a definitive diagnosis in a very young child.

What Are the Signs and Symptoms of Primary Headaches in Children?

MIGRAINE

Migraine is defined by the presence of recurrent attacks of moderate to severe headache with throbbing or pulsatile quality that worsens with activity. Pain is accompanied by nausea, vomiting, or sensitivity to light and sound. Observation of these symptoms is sufficient, even if the child does not report them. Migraine headaches in children can be bilateral (whereas the pain is usually unilateral in adults) and without treatment the pain may last 2 hours or longer (the pain usually lasts at least 4 hours in adults). Relief upon falling asleep as well as the desire to fall asleep are very common complaints in prepubescent migraineurs, and may be a central feature of these headaches.

Migraine can be accompanied by reversible visual, sensory, speech, motor, brainstem, or retinal symptoms, called aura; these symptoms usually evolve over a few minutes and are accompanied by or followed within 60 minutes by headache. Classically, visual phenomena in migraine include a flickering, zigzag-shaped spreading blurring of the field of vision (scintillating scotoma). Children may also experience a distortion in the size and distance to objects ("Alice in Wonderland" syndrome). Visual auras preceding a headache are much less common before the age of 10.[8] Prolonged migraines that last longer than 3 days are called status migrainosus. When these headaches occur very frequently for a long time (at least 15 days per month for at least 3 months), the term *chronic migraine* is used. Of note, many patients who have migraine also have tension-type headaches.

TENSION-TYPE HEADACHE

These headaches are bilateral, of mild to moderate intensity, with a pressing or tight quality. The pain is not usually made worse by activity, and does not have associated symptoms like nausea, vomiting, nor sensitivity to light and sound. The pain can last from minutes to days. Most people experience some tension-type headaches at some point in their life without significant problem, but frequent tension-type headaches can be disabling. When these headaches occur very frequently for a long time (at least 15 days per month for at least 3 months), the term *chronic tension-type headache* is used.

Primary Stabbing Headache

This pain, also called ice pick headache, usually lasts less than 3 seconds but can last up to a few minutes. The pain may recur one to several times per day, and often comes at irregular intervals. The pain may occur at a consistent spot on the head or may move around the head and is associated with a brief facial grimace. The presence of autonomic symptoms with the pain or consistent location of the pain should prompt evaluation for another etiology.

Trigeminal Autonomic Cephalgias

These are very uncommon in children. Headaches in this category include short-lasting unilateral neuralgiform headache attacks with conjunctival injection and tearing (SUNCT), paroxysmal hemicrania, cluster headache, and hemicrania continua. These headaches usually occur on only one side of the head, and are accompanied by same-side autonomic symptoms, including excessive lacrimation, nasal discharge, or drooping eyelid. The primary differences between these entities are in the frequencies and duration. Hemicrania continua is nearly continuous for months, cluster headache lasts minutes to hours, paroxysmal hemicrania lasts minutes, and SUNCT lasts seconds. Hemicrania continua and paroxysmal hemicrania respond well to indomethacin, whereas cluster headaches acutely respond to oxygen.[8]

Periodic Syndromes of Childhood

These include cyclic vomiting, abdominal migraine, benign paroxysmal vertigo, alternating hemiplegia, and benign paroxysmal torticollis, which are addressed elsewhere in the book. These conditions share many qualities with migraine, but in each of these the primary symptom is something other than pain in the head.

Summary

The central role of a general pediatrician in managing headache is in the identification and treatment of causes of secondary headache. The use of the SNOOPY mnemonic may aid in differentiating these from primary headache syndromes. Treatment depends on the specific headache type, with chronic primary headache syndromes most amenable to management by pediatric neurologists.

References

1. Mortimer MJ, Kay J, Jaron A. Epidemiology of headache and childhood migraine in an urban general practice using Ad Hoc, Vahlquist and IHS criteria. *Dev Med Child Neurol.* 1992;34(12):1095-1101.
2. Lateef TM, Merikangas KR, He J, et al. Headache in a national sample of American children: prevalence and comorbidity. *J Child Neurol.* 2009;24(5):536-543.
3. Schobitz E, Qureshi F, Lewis D. Pediatric headaches in the emergency department. *Curr Pain Headache Rep.* 2006;10(5):391-396.
4. Kernick D, Stapley S, Campbell J, Hamilton W. What happens to new-onset headache in children that present to primary care? A case-cohort study using electronic primary care records. *Cephalalgia.* 2009;29(12):1311-1316.
5. Raieli V, Eliseo M, Pandolfi E, et al. Recurrent and chronic headaches in children below 6 years of age. *J Headache Pain.* 2005;6(3):135-142.
6. Dodick DW. Pearls: headache. *Semin Neurol.* 2010;30(1):74-81.
7. Lewis DW, Ashwal S, Dahl G, et al. Practice parameter: evaluation of children and adolescents with recurrent headaches: report of the Quality Standards Subcommittee of the American Academy of Neurology and the Practice Committee of the Child Neurology Society. *Neurology.* 2002;59(4):490-498.
8. Headache Classification Committee of the International Headache Society. The International Classification of Headache Disorders. 3rd ed (beta version). *Cephalalgia.* 2013;33(9):629-808.

WHEN SHOULD I CONSIDER HEAD IMAGING IN A CHILD WITH HEADACHE? COMPUTED TOMOGRAPHY OR MAGNETIC RESONANCE IMAGING?

Laura A. Adang, MD, PhD

Headache is a common complaint in pediatric patients and most often has a benign cause or is due to a primary headache syndrome. The worry of most parents who bring their child for headache evaluation is, does my child have a brain tumor? It is, therefore, crucial to distinguish the benign headache from those with a secondary and usually more concerning cause, such as trauma, infection, tumor, or stroke. However, not every patient with a headache needs head imaging. Both computed tomography (CT) and magnetic resonance imaging (MRI) impart some risk to the child, and it is rare that neuroimaging findings will change the management of a patient with a normal neurological exam. A recent meta-analysis found that imaging findings changed management in only 3% of patients in whom head imaging was performed and there was an exam abnormality in all patients who required surgical treatment.[1] So how do we decide? I typically start with a broad differential for causes of headache and use the history and physical exam to look for red flags that may indicate a more sinister diagnosis. The initial goal of the headache consultation is to determine: does this child need additional evaluation or is this clearly a benign or primary headache?

A detailed headache history is the first step in distinguishing primary headache syndromes from secondary headaches. When did the pain start and has it worsened over time? Has the child experienced a headache like this before? How often do the headaches occur? Where is it located and does it radiate? How severe is the pain? What makes it better or worse? Does it worsen with exertion and improve with rest? Does it wake the child in the middle of the night? Is it accompanied by nausea, vomiting, photophobia, or phonophobia? Is there any visual change with the headache, such as sparkling lights? Are there any associated neurologic symptoms like weakness, numbness, or dizziness? Is there a family history of headache or migraine? Additionally, a thorough review of systems helps to elucidate any associated symptoms, such as visual or auditory changes, neurologic symptoms, weight loss, night sweats, fevers, drug or toxin exposures (including carbon

Licht DJ, Ryan NR, eds. *Curbside Consultation in Pediatric Neurology: 49 Clinical Questions* (pp 81-83).
© 2016 Taylor & Francis Group.

Table 17-1
Headache Red Flags

- History
  - Change from typical headache pattern
  - Thunderclap onset or "worst headache of life"
  - Worse in the middle of the night or first thing in the morning
  - Occipital location
  - Immunocompromised state
  - Neurologic signs or symptoms (including seizures, altered mental status)
  - Recent head or neck injury
  - Triggered by Valsalva maneuvers (coughing, straining)
  - No family history
  - Young age (< 3)
- Exam
  - Fever or signs of infection
  - Nuchal rigidity
  - Signs of increased intracranial pressure (eye movement abnormalities, papilledema)
  - Macrocephaly
  - Focal neurologic signs (weakness, sensory change)

---

monoxide), and rashes (for infectious causes such as Lyme disease). Another factor to consider is the age of the child and whether he or she can give an adequate headache history. While there are no clear guidelines, I typically image any child complaining of headache under the age of 3 years.

The next step is a comprehensive neurologic examination, including head circumference, visual acuity, visualization of the optic discs, and blood pressure measurement. If the optic discs are not well visualized, the child should be referred for a dilated exam. Many of these headache "red flags" on history and physical are listed in Table 17-1. In one study, the most salient predictors of a cause that required surgical intervention were headache of less than 1 month duration, no family history of migraine, abnormal neurologic findings on examination, gait abnormality, and occurrence of seizures. The presence of a red flag prompts a need for imaging and indicates the urgency with which that imaging is needed.[1]

Certain findings on history or physical exam may suggest a particular secondary cause. For example, while there are no headache characteristics unique to brain tumors, these headaches are frequently associated with other symptoms and are usually chronic and progressively worsening, evolving over weeks to months. Any signs of possible increased intracranial pressure, such as papilledema, nocturnal or early morning awakenings with vomiting, and worsening with the Valsalva maneuver are concerning and thus neuroimaging should be considered as this suggests an intracranial mass. Posterior fossa tumors, in particular, can present with occipital, progressive headaches.

The presence of malaise, fever, or a stiff neck (meningismus) raises the concern for an intracranial infection, such as meningitis or abscess. Once the patient is stable and on appropriate antibiotics, I obtain a head MRI to investigate for abscesses, sinus extension, or signs of emboli for a systemic source, such as an infected cardiac valve. Lyme disease in children can present with headache, although rarely as an isolated symptom. Any immunocompromised patient should have both head imaging and a lumbar puncture given the increased risk of severe infection.

Children, like adults, can have vascular causes of their headaches, including hypertension and arterial dissections, and these headaches need further imaging evaluation. Dissections commonly present with a severe, constant, ipsilateral headache, and neck pain. To determine the likelihood, I ask about other risk factors including Ehlers-Danlos and Marfan syndromes, infections, coughing, neck trauma, and recent activities (like riding a roller coaster). With any focal neurologic signs such a Horner's or suspicious history, I consider imaging the cerebral vasculature as well.

If there are red flags on history or exam, the question then becomes, should a head CT or MRI of the brain be ordered? For a child who needs urgent or emergent imaging, noncontrast head CT is usually preferable. This can be performed quickly, in most cases, without needing to sedate a child and is readily available in the emergency department. I use head CTs for any headache patient with a possible vascular etiology, recent trauma, signs of increased intracranial pressure, or a focal neurologic finding on exam for which imaging may change immediate management. One such concerning feature on history suggesting a vascular etiology is the sudden "thunderclap" headache, which can be caused by hemorrhage, cerebral venous sinus thrombosis, dissection, and vasospasm. Head CT does involve exposure to radiation, which is particularly concerning for the pediatric patient; however, this risk is minimal in a child who has not had frequent CT scans and radiation exposure is limited when contrast is not used.

MRI imaging is superior for characterizing headaches from infections and tumors, particularly in the posterior fossa. There is no radiation involved but the study takes longer to perform than a head CT. Most children under the age of 6 and many above this age will need sedation in order to lie still for an MRI. While sedation is generally safe, it does introduce risk for breathing issues or reactions to medication during the procedure. For the vast majority of cases, gadolinium contrast is not needed for the initial evaluation of headache although it is safe in the pediatric population. Contrast administration also increases the duration of the study leading to a longer sedation time. MRI can be considered when red flags are present but there are no emergent indicators for head imaging as described above.

The headaches of most children have a benign etiology and do not need further imaging or evaluation. Using a thorough, tailored history and a physical examination, particularly focused on the neurologic components, we can easily determine which patients need head imaging.

Reference

1. Abend NS, Younkin D, Lewis DW. Secondary headaches in children and adolescents. *Semin in Pediatr Neurol.* 2010;17:123-133.

Suggested Readings

DeLuca GC, Bartleson JD. When and how to investigate the patient with headache. *Semin in Pediatr Neurol.* 2010;30:131-144.

Lewis DW, Ashwal S, Dahl G, et al. Practice parameter: evaluation of children and adolescents with recurrent headaches. *Neurology.* 2002;59:490-498.

WHAT MEDICATIONS ARE BEST TO ABORT A MIGRAINE?

Steven Kugler, MD

Migraine headaches are the most common primary headache in children. They occur with increasing frequency through adolescence. The reported prevalence increases from 3% (age 3 to 7 years) to 4% to 11% (ages 7 to 11) to 8% to 23% (ages 11 to 15 +). The mean age of onset is 7.2 years for boys and 10.9 years for girls. Migraine headaches are a frequent presentation to the pediatrician's office and emergency department (ED). Migraines are both underdiagnosed and I consider undertreated.

The present classification criteria for migraine diagnosis uses the 2004 *International Criteria for Headache Disorders, Second Edition*. Migraine headaches can be different in children and adolescents as compared to their adult counterparts. The duration of attack can be shorter, pain can be bilateral, photophobia and phonophobia may not occur together, aura symptoms are less common, and gastrointestinal symptoms are more prominent. Younger children often have difficulty articulating their symptoms, and I often must rely on behavioral manifestations observed by their parents.

The goal of abortive therapy of pediatric migraine should be a quick response with return to normal activity without relapse. Attacks should be treated rapidly and consistently. A medication should have a high tolerability with minimal side effects. Medications should be administered as early as possible in the progression of the migraine. Especially in children, appropriate doses should be given in accordance with the child's age and weight. Medications should be limited to avoid overuse headache. For me, an important component in the management of pediatric migraine is education of the patient and parents.

In the pharmacological treatment of acute migraine in children and adolescents, there remains a paucity of positive controlled clinical studies in the literature. One of the main reasons is the high placebo response rate in children. As such we are often compelled to extrapolate from the adult experience.

Licht DJ, Ryan NR, eds. *Curbside Consultation in Pediatric Neurology: 49 Clinical Questions* (pp 85-87).
© 2016 Taylor & Francis Group.

At the onset of a migraine, I emphasize to patients the importance of drinking at least 8 to 16 ounces (0.2 to 0.5 L) of fluid as they take their medication. Over-the-counter medications are the mainstay of acute treatment, particularly in young children. There is more than ample evidence in controlled studies to confirm the efficacy of acetaminophen and ibuprofen. Recommended doses are acetaminophen at 15 mg/kg/dose and ibuprofen 10 mg/kg/dose. Naproxen, although less studied, can also be used at a dose of 5 to 10 mg/kg/dose. Aspirin use in adults has been found to be effective and is often taken. Aspirin in pediatrics is usually reserved for older adolescents because of the concerns of developing Reye's syndrome in the context of a febrile illness or metabolic disorder. In the use of these over-the-counter medications, one should be concerned about overuse headache and rebound. I typically limit their use to 2 to 3 times per week if possible. I generally avoid opiates in the outpatient treatment of childhood migraine.

The triptans have gained widespread use in the adult population since the introduction of sumatriptan in the United States in 1993. This class of medications includes serotonin 1B/1D agonists and have been a major advance in abortive therapy. The triptans are considered to be migraine-specific agents and can be used when a patient fails a more general nonsteroidal anti-inflammatory drug (NSAID) or acetaminophen. Almotriptan has been approved by the Food and Drug Administration for use in adolescents (12 to 17 years) and rizatriptan is approved for 6- to 17-year-old patients. I commonly use these and the other triptans in my pediatric patients. While multiple studies have demonstrated the efficacy of the other triptans in children and adolescents, there have also been conflicting results. The triptans most studied to date in pediatrics have been sumatriptan, almotriptan, rizatriptan, and zolmitriptan. My selection of a specific triptan often depends on the mode of delivery and whether nausea and vomiting are present. Some children cannot swallow pills and either a nasal formulation or orally disintegrating tablet may be best. Sumatriptan comes as a subcutaneous form (4 mg, 6 mg), oral tablet (25 mg, 50 mg, 100 mg), and nasal spray (5 mg, 20 mg). Sumatriptan nasal spray may have the most promising data, with its main side effect being a bad taste. Almotriptan comes in 6.25-mg and 12.5-mg tablets. Rizatriptan comes as a tablet (5 mg, 10 mg) and also an orally dissolving tablet. Zolmitriptan comes as a tablet (2.5 mg, 5 mg), oral disintegrating tablet (2.5 mg, 5 mg), and a nasal spray (2.5 mg, 5 mg). I usually limit triptan use to 2 days per week. An appropriate dose for a triptan is not clearly weight related. I find that if one triptan is ineffective, it does not preclude the trial of another triptan that may be effective. Triptans are contraindicated in children with prior stroke, cardiovascular disease, hypertension, and hemiplegic migraine. They can be used in migraine with aura. Side effects include worsening headache, flushing, nausea, chest pain, dizziness, and fatigue.

Combination therapy using an NSAID and a triptan has been effectively used in adults. In one large pediatric placebo-controlled study, the combination of sumatriptan and naproxen showed superiority. The combination of an NSAID and a triptan may be a reasonable option for those who have partial relief with the use of an NSAID or triptan alone. Other NSAIDs available include oral ketorolac and diclofenac sodium. Intranasal dihydroergotamine can be used as abortive therapy but there are limited pediatric data.

In the adjunctive treatment of migraine, antiemetics in either the suppository or oral forms can be used in children with acute migraine that is accompanied by nausea or vomiting. Promethazine, prochlorperazine, and metoclopramide can be quite effective and may also show therapeutic effect against the migraine itself. I also use ondansetron, which doesn't have the risk of extrapyramidal side effects, but treats only the nausea and vomiting.

Children and adolescents present to the ED when acute therapies at home have failed or they have entered into status migrainosus. Most patients have already tried a migraine-abortive medication before their arrival to the ED. There is a lack of controlled trials of pediatric migraine patients treated in the ED. As such, protocols vary greatly among institutions. At our hospital, the ED management may often advance to parenteral medications depending on what was tried at home, the severity, and duration of the migraine. Children with migraine may have vomiting before their ED arrival and their oral intake may have been poor secondary to nausea. Hydration can be accomplished by an intravenous (IV) normal saline bolus of 20 cc/kg. Ensuring good hydration may also provide renal protection before treatment with an NSAID such as ketorolac because higher doses of ketorolac can be associated with acute renal failure. For analgesia, we often use IV ketorolac at 0.5 mg/kg/dose every 6 hours with a maximum of 30 mg/dose. We prefer IV metoclopramide at 0.2 mg/kg/dose with a maximum of 20 mg/dose as an antiemetic and also for treating the migraine head pain.

In the ED if hydration, ketorolac, and metoclopramide are not effective, we advance to second-line therapy. Valproate IV at 15 mg/kg to a maximum of 1000 mg has been found to be effective. Prior to the use of valproate in females, a negative pregnancy test needs to be obtained. If the IV valproate is effective, we may discharge the patient on oral valproate if prophylactic medication is indicated. Another option in the ED is IV steroids, which we have found to be helpful. We often use IV methylprednisolone at 2 mg/kg to a maximum of 200 mg. There is evidence that a single dose of steroids may decrease the likelihood of headache recurrence. If our migraine patient still has not gained relief, then inpatient treatment is warranted. Approaches could include IV dihydroergotamine, magnesium, or levetiracetam.

If a child has become headache free at the time of ED discharge, then a plan should be instituted to provide adequate tools at home to treat the next migraine attack effectively. The objective would be to treat the next migraine successfully at home and avoid an ED revisit.

Over the years much progress has been made in the abortive treatment of pediatric migraine, particularly with the introduction of migraine-specific medications. In the pharmacological treatment of migraine we need to balance medication phobia and medication overuse. Finally, in the management of pediatric migraine a treatment plan should be implemented that addresses the specific needs of the child or adolescent.

Suggested Readings

Derosier FJ, Lewis D, Hershey A, et al. Randomized trial of sumatriptan and naproxen sodium combination in adolescent migraine. *Pediatrics.* 2012;129(6):e1411-e1420.

Gelfand A, Goadsby P. Treatment of pediatric migraine in the emergency room. *Pediatr Neurol.* 2012;47(4):233-241.

Hershey AD. Current approaches to the diagnosis and management of pediatric migraine. *Lancet Neurol.* 2010;9:190-204.

Lewis D, Ashwal S, Hershey A, Hirtz D, Yonker M, Silberstein S. Practice parameter: pharmacological treatment of migraine headache in children and adolescents. *Neurology.* 2004;63(12):2215-2224.

Pakalnis A. Current therapies in childhood and adolescent migraine. *J Child Neurol.* 2007;22(11):1288-1292.

Vollono C, Vigevano F, Tarantino S, Valeriani M. Triptans other than sumatriptan in child and adolescent migraine: literature review. *Expert Rev Neurother.* 2011;11(3):395-401.

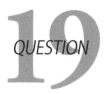

ARE THERE WAYS TO PREVENT MIGRAINES? WHAT LIFESTYLE FACTORS CONTRIBUTE TO HEADACHES?

Christina Szperka, MD and Emily Robbins, MD

Migraine is usually an episodic disorder, though a small percentage of patients report very frequent or even constant headache. Though there are several medications that can effectively treat the acute symptoms, when possible it is better to prevent the attacks. Prevention includes 2 approaches: lifestyle modifications and, for patients with frequent or disabling headaches, preventive medications.

Lifestyle Factors

Migraineurs have a hyperexcitable brain, more prone to react and overreact to stimuli. Fluctuations in sleeping, eating, and hydration patterns can trigger attacks, so good self-care can help to reduce a patient's headache frequency. Most of the following "healthy habits" are common sense, and applicable to anyone, but are particularly important for migraineurs.

- Get enough sleep: Children with migraine headaches have more sleep disturbances, including longer sleep onset delay, more resistance to bedtime, greater sleep anxiety, shorter sleep duration, more nighttime awakenings, more parasomnias, more sleep-disordered breathing, and more daytime sleepiness, than those without migraines.[1] Patients should get enough sleep so that they do not feel tired, usually 8 to 10 hours per night, with no daytime naps. If it is necessary to rest to treat a headache, that should be limited to 15 minutes to avoid disruption of the sleep cycle. It is important to follow a consistent schedule, going to sleep and getting up at the same time each day, varying from day to day by an hour or less. Attention to sleep hygiene can help, including avoidance of stimulating activities such as electronics and homework in bed.

Licht DJ, Ryan NR, eds. *Curbside Consultation in Pediatric Neurology: 49 Clinical Questions* (pp 89-93).
© 2016 Taylor & Francis Group.

Table 19-1
Recommended Fluid Intake by Weight

Weight in Pounds	Minimum Amount/Day	
	Number of Ounces	*Number of 8-Ounce Cups*
40 to 60	48	6
60 to 80	56	7
80 to 100	64	8
100 to 120	72	9
120 to 140	80	10
140 to 160	88	11
160 to 180	96	12
180 to 200	104	13

- Drink more fluid: Most people do not drink enough fluid to maintain normal hydration. Increased headache with exercise can be a sign of dehydration. See Table 19-1 for recommended fluid intake. Most of the fluid should be water. Soda and juice have empty calories that can cause weight gain, which will worsen headaches and cause other health problems. Caffeine should be minimized because it acts as a diuretic. If necessary, write a letter to allow patients to carry a water bottle in school to maintain adequate hydration throughout the day. Children should drink extra fluid before and during exercise and immediately at onset of headache.

- Eat regularly: Skipping meals, fasting, and low blood sugar can trigger migraines. Encourage all children, particularly teenagers, to eat breakfast every morning, provide snacks as needed throughout the day, and eat well-balanced meals with protein and fiber to avoid dramatic shifts in blood sugar.

- Eat foods that help prevent migraines: Low levels of certain vitamins and minerals may contribute to migraines and fatigue, so it is important to eat dark green vegetables and whole grains for vitamin B_2 and magnesium, vitamin-D fortified dairy products or soy milk, and lean meat, fish, beans, or nuts for coenzyme Q10.

- Watch foods that can trigger headaches: Encourage the patient or parents to keep a log of what was eaten in the 12 to 24 hours before a migraine attack to see whether the removal or reduction of certain foods from the diet improves headaches. Specific foods to watch:

  ○ Caffeine: Withdrawal from caffeine can trigger a headache. Limit caffeinated soda, iced tea, coffee, and energy drinks to 3 days/week.

  ○ Monosodium glutamate: This is a common food additive in prepared, canned, and frozen foods. It can also be called yeast extract, hydrolyzed vegetable protein, automated yeast, sodium caseinate, and texturized protein.

  ○ Alcohol: Many teenagers have experimented with alcohol. It may be a trigger even if not openly acknowledged.

○ Many people worry about foods like chocolate, aged cheese, cured meats, and peanut butter, though there is some evidence that these dietary triggers are overemphasized. If any of those foods are triggers for headaches, patients should avoid them. It may be helpful to remove all worrisome foods from the diet for a few weeks, then add back one food every few days to see if it affects the headache. If none of those foods trigger headaches, they may be consumed in moderation.

- Exercise: Exercise triggers the body to release anti-pain chemicals, aids sleep, decreases stress, and helps to control weight. Children should perform aerobic exercise a minimum of 30 minutes 3 times/week. Many children with chronic headache report that their pain increases with activity. Using the headache as a guide, advise patients that it is not dangerous to exercise until the pain increases slightly, as repeatedly exercising to this threshold can increase tolerance and decrease pain over time.

- Identify and reduce stress: Stress can trigger headaches. Advise patients to think carefully about home, school, and social life. Teach them that good stress (like preparing for a party) and stress let-down (crashing after a big event) can also be triggers for headaches. Studies have shown that a combination of medication and stress reduction therapy works better than either one by itself to improve headaches.[2] Consider one of the following:

  ○ Relaxation training: Relaxation training includes techniques such as progressive muscle relaxation, breathing exercises, and guided imagery. These techniques are best suited for children ages 7 and older but can be modified for younger children and those with intellectual disabilities.[3,4]

  ○ Biofeedback: Biofeedback is a way of training the mind to provide relaxation and decrease pain, and is usually taught by psychologists. The goal of biofeedback is for the patient to learn to identify and actively change a physiologic function. To do this, the physiologic function is given a visual or auditory representation that can be consciously perceived by the individual, and then adjusted.[4] For patients with headache, electromyographic (EMG) activity is used as a correlate of muscle tension, and skin temperature is used as a correlate of the vasomotor mechanisms. By providing patients with a visual display of these measurements, children can become aware of their bodies' physical responses and then learn to control these responses through relaxation.[3]

  ○ Cognitive behavioral therapy (CBT): CBT is another type of therapy taught by psychologists. CBT focuses on finding ways to change a person's response to pain and stress. In CBT the patient learns to correlate his or her thoughts and behaviors with the body's reactions, and then employs strategies to modify those thoughts and behaviors.[4]

- Identify comorbid psychological problems: Children want to know what causes their headache, what can make it better, and whether they are going to die as a result.[5] Providers can ease that anxiety by providing an explanation for the pain, a treatment plan, and reassurance. The pain of the headache itself, as well as the concomitant interruption in everyday life, can lead to anxiety and depression. Providers should screen for anxiety and depression using validated scales and treat accordingly.[3]

- Keep a diary to figure out triggers: Keeping a headache diary is the best way to recognize what triggers the headache. Advise patients to keep track of the following:

  ○ Headaches (including severity)

  ○ Medicines (acute and preventive)

  ○ Possible triggers (changes in sleep schedule, foods)

  ○ Menstrual cycle

Preventive Medications

When lifestyle modifications fail to reduce migraine frequency to fewer than 4 days per month or the patient misses significant time from school, pharmacological prevention should be initiated. The goal in using preventive medications is to reduce headache frequency and/or severity by 50%. To minimize side effects, increase dose slowly over a few weeks, and continue the medication at the goal dose for 2 months before deciding whether it has been beneficial. If no benefit, wean the medication off over 1 to 2 weeks and start another preventive medication (cross-tapering is sometimes appropriate). If the medication has been helpful, continue it until the patient has had 6 months of well-controlled headaches once per week or less often, and then slowly taper off the medication.

Many medications have been used, but there are very few high-quality studies of the efficacy of these drugs in children. Most studies have been open-label observational case series, and interpretation is limited by the high placebo rate in pediatric headache, patient and dose heterogeneity, and short duration. Because of the limited data, there is no standard approach to preventive medications. Multiple classes of drugs can be used to prevent migraines, including antidepressants, antiserotonergic, antiepileptics, and antihypertensives. Below is specific information about the ones we use most commonly:

- Antidepressants: Amitriptyline (up to 1 mg/kg/day) has been shown to be effective in a number of open-label studies. This is the first choice of many providers for older children and adolescents. It is dosed once daily near bedtime, and also treats insomnia. Because tricyclics can cause QT prolongation, check an electrocardiogram prior to starting amitriptyline, and again at 1 mg/kg/day. Other than sedation, the main side effects are dry eyes, dry mouth, and constipation.

- Antiserotonergic: Cyproheptadine (up to 0.25 to 0.3 mg/kg/day) has positive evidence from an open-label study and has been used for many years. This is the first choice of many providers when treating headaches in young children because it is an old medicine for allergies, comes in a liquid formulation, and can be dosed 1 to 2 times per day. It can help to treat comorbid gastrointestinal complaints, and stimulates the appetite.

- Antiepileptics:
  - Topiramate is the best studied among the preventive medications, with multiple randomized, double-blind, placebo-controlled studies showing a statistically significant decrease in migraine days per month and decreased disability when compared to placebo.[6-8] Topiramate (up to 2 mg/kg/day) is given twice daily, and unlike most migraine preventives it does not cause weight gain. However, it commonly causes sedation, tingling in the hands and feet, belly upset, and cognitive side effects, and less commonly causes decreased sweating, kidney stones, and glaucoma. Topiramate also interferes with birth control pills, making them less effective, and is teratogenic.

  - Valproic acid is also supported by multiple studies and can also treat comorbid psychiatric disease, but its use in adolescent female migraineurs is limited by its side effect profile, including weight gain, association with ovarian cysts, and teratogenicity.

There are also many supplements that have been shown to decrease headache frequency. See Table 19-2.

While these interventions require significant investment of time on the part of providers and families, empowering children to engage in behaviors that prevent headaches will have long-lasting benefits.

Table 19-2
Supplements for Headache Prevention

Supplement	Starting Dose	Special Considerations
Riboflavin	Up to 6 years: 50 mg bid 6 to 8 years: 100 mg bid 8 to 13 years: 150 mg bid 13 years+: 200 mg bid	• Found in dark, leafy green vegetables and whole grains • Will turn urine yellow-green or yellow-orange • Take with food
Magnesium	Start with 250 mg of magnesium oxide once daily, can increase up to 250 mg tid Magnesium dosing for other forms: 0.5 to 0.75 mEq/kg/day in 3 to 4 divided doses	• Found in green vegetables, some legumes, and whole grains • Side effects: diarrhea, bad taste • Do not use in patients with severe renal failure
Coenzyme Q10	100 mg in the morning, can increase as needed up to 3 mg/day	• Helpful in headache and fatigue • Side effects: stomach upset, insomnia

Not recommended due to insufficient data: feverfew, Tenoten (antibodies to brain-specific protein S100B), L-carnitine, ginkgolide B, melatonin.
Not recommended due to safety concerns: butterbur.

bid: twice/day; tid: 3 times/day.

References

1. Miller VA, Palermo TM, Powers SW, Scher MS, Hershey AD. Migraine headaches and sleep disturbances in children. *Headache*. 2003;43(4):362-368.
2. Powers SW, Kashikar-Zuck SM, Allen JR, et al. Cognitive behavioral therapy plus amitriptyline for chronic migraine in children and adolescents: a randomized clinical trial. *JAMA*. 2013;310(24):2622-2630.
3. Powers SW, Andrasik F. Biobehavioral treatment, disability, and psychological effects of pediatric headache. *Pediatr Ann*. 2005;34(6):461-465.
4. Kropp P, Meyer B, Landgraf M, Ruscheweyh R, Ebinger F, Straube A. Headache in children: update on biobehavioral treatments. *Neuropediatrics*. 2013;44(1):20-24.
5. Lewis DW, Middlebrook MT, Mehallick L, Rauch TM, Deline C, Thomas EF. Pediatric headaches: what do the children want? *Headache*. 1996;36(4):224-230.
6. Lakshmi CV, Singhi P, Malhi P, Ray M. Topiramate in the prophylaxis of pediatric migraine: a double-blind placebo-controlled trial. *J Child Neurol*. 2007;22(7):829-835.
7. Winner P, Gendolla A, Stayer C, et al. Topiramate for migraine prevention in adolescents: a pooled analysis of efficacy and safety. *Headache*. 2006;46(10):1503-1510.
8. Lewis D, Winner P, Saper J, et al. Randomized, double-blind, placebo-controlled study to evaluate the efficacy and safety of topiramate for migraine prevention in pediatric subjects 12 to 17 years of age. *Pediatrics*. 2009;123(3):924-934.

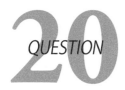

ARE TENSION-TYPE HEADACHES TREATED DIFFERENTLY FROM MIGRAINES?

Joyce Sapin, MD

According to the current classification system for tension-type headaches (TTH) established by the International Headache Society in 2004,[1] TTH last from 30 minutes to 7 days. The pain has at least 2 of the following characteristics: bilateral location, pressure/tightening (nonpulsating) quality, mild or moderate intensity, and the headache is not aggravated by routine physical activity. Additionally there is no associated nausea or vomiting and there is either light or sound sensitivity but not both. In comparison, migraine headaches may be preceded by an aura and are usually unilateral, pulsating, aggravated by physical activity, and associated with nausea/vomiting, photophobia, and phonophobia. Features of migraines and tension headaches often overlap. Some days headaches may resemble TTH and on other days a migraine headache. Migraines seem to be more disabling than TTH. TTH are often more commonly associated with muscle pain and tension, in particular at the back of the head/neck and shoulders. As younger children in particular often have difficulty describing their symptoms, at times I find it difficult to differentiate between the 2 types of headaches (Table 20-1).

Following a detailed history, a thorough physical and neurological examination is performed. Atypical symptoms in the history such as nocturnal headaches that waken the patient from sleep, recurrent focal headaches, headaches associated with Valsalva maneuvers, and persistent vomiting are concerning. Abnormalities on examination such as asymmetric reflexes, abnormal funduscopic examination, nuchal rigidity, and unsteady gait are also "red flags" that should prompt further testing to evaluate for serious secondary causes of headaches (see Question 17). Additional studies may include laboratory tests, neuroimaging, and possibly cerebrospinal fluid examination.

Although therapy involves both nonpharmacological and pharmacological modalities, my first line of treatment both for TTH and migraines is nonpharmacological. I recommend starting a headache diary to monitor various triggers. This includes sleep pattern/sleep hygiene, dietary factors, menstruation, barometric pressure changes, and psychosocial stressors both at home and

Licht DJ, Ryan NR, eds. *Curbside Consultation in Pediatric Neurology: 49 Clinical Questions* (pp 95-98).
© 2016 Taylor & Francis Group.

Table 20-1

Similarities and Differences Between Tension-Type Headaches and Migraines

	Tension-Type Headaches	Migraines
Location and quality of pain	Bilateral Pressure tightening Nonpulsating	More commonly unilateral Pulsating
Intensity	Mild or moderate	Moderate or severe
	Not aggravated by physical activity	Aggravated by physical activity
Associated symptoms	No nausea/vomiting Light or sound sensitivity, not both	± Aura Nausea/vomiting Light and sound sensitivity
Muscle pain	In particular at the back of the head/neck and shoulders	Not usually present
Frequency	More common school days	Both school days and school breaks
Comorbid conditions	Anxiety/depression	Anxiety/depression
First line of treatment	Eliminate triggers Counseling/biofeedback	Eliminate triggers Counseling/biofeedback
First-line pharmacologic treatment	Over-the-counter analgesics NSAIDs May consider Fioricet	Over-the-counter analgesics NSAIDs Fioricet
Second-line pharmacologic treatment	Antiemetics on occasion	Antiemetics Triptans
Preventive medication	Tricyclic antidepressants Beta blockers Anticonvulsants	Tricyclic antidepressants Beta blockers Anticonvulsants
Cofactors	Magnesium Riboflavin	Magnesium Riboflavin

NSAIDs: nonsteroidal anti-inflammatory drugs.

school. It is important for patients and parents (when dealing with younger children) to try to determine possible precipitants. In my experience, TTH headaches are more common on school days and seem to improve on weekends and school holidays/breaks. Migraines are often seen both during school and school breaks. Among adolescents in particular, both types of headaches seem to be increased in those with comorbid conditions such as anxiety and depression.

Identified triggers need to be addressed and modified if possible. This might include eliminating electronics at night, not napping after school, and trying not to sleep too late on weekends. Regular and nutritious meals are important, including eating breakfast on school days and limiting caffeine intake. Increased fluid consumption, in particular water during the day, is helpful as is regular aerobic exercise. Counseling is often beneficial in developing coping skills to deal with psychosocial stressors, especially in individuals with comorbid conditions such as depression and anxiety. Other nonpharmacological treatments that I often recommend include relaxation/biofeedback techniques, cognitive behavior therapy, hypnosis, stress reducers such as massage and yoga, and even acupuncture/acupressure.

Pharmacological treatment both for TTH and migraines includes abortive medication (at onset of symptoms) and preventive or prophylactic medication (to prevent frequent symptoms). In both TTH and migraines, I first suggest administration of over-the-counter analgesics such as ibuprofen, acetaminophen, and naproxen. The correct dose for weight should be reviewed. The use of analgesics needs to be limited to prevent rebound headaches as well as medication-overuse headaches. I also use over-the-counter analgesics in conjunction with Benadryl (diphenhydramine). If these are ineffective, the next line of treatment I prescribe is either prescription nonsteroidal anti-inflammatory drugs and/or Fioricet (butalbital, acetaminophen, and caffeine). In my practice, I do not prescribe triptans for typical TTH that do not progress to migraines. Antiemetics are used more frequently for migraines. I use these agents in patients with TTH who also have migraines and may develop nausea from the use of analgesics.

If TTH are becoming chronic (>15 days per month for >3 months) and resulting in missed school days, I prescribe preventive treatment. The prophylactic medications that I use are similar to those agents used for migraine headaches and include tricyclic antidepressants, beta blockers, and anticonvulsants. I start with the lowest dose and titrate slowly to minimize side effects. I usually continue medication for several months. If the patient is doing well I attempt to slowly wean the medication, preferably at the end of the school year. I also recommend cofactors such as magnesium and riboflavin, which seem to improve symptoms both in TTH and migraines. Both vitamin D and iron deficiency have been associated with TTH and migraines. Supplements of both if levels are low have been beneficial.

Although the pathophysiology as well as the definition of TTH and migraines is different, many patients often experience both types of headaches either concurrently or at different times. In the pediatric population, our patients often have difficulty defining pain, making it difficult to discern the 2 types of headaches. In my opinion the evaluation and nonpharmacologic treatment both for TTH and migraines are similar. Abortive medication may differ slightly with regard to the use of triptans but preventive medication prescribed for both is often the same. A multifaceted plan is essential in order for successful resolution of symptoms both in TTH and migraines.

Reference

1. Headache Classification Subcommittee of the International Headache Society. The International Classification of Headache Disorders. 2nd ed. *Cephalalgia.* 2004;24(Suppl 1):9-160.

Suggested Readings

Blume HK. Pediatric headache: a review. *Pediatr Rev.* 2012;33(12):562-576.

Parisi P, Papetti L, Spalice A, Nicita F, Ursitti F, Villa MP. Tension-type headache in paediatric age. *Acta Paediatr.* 2011;100(4):491-495.

What Is a "Migraine Variant"? Is It Treated Differently?

Daniel J. Licht, MD

Migraine variant (or *migraine equivalent*) is the term applied to a migraine that exhibits itself in a form other than cephalgia (head pain) alone. Such conditions are less recognized, less common, and indeed less well understood than the typical migraines (both without and with aura) that usually affect children and young adults. The *International Classification of Headache Disorders, Second Edition* has, in part, confused the terminology by doing away with the term *migraine variant* in favor of a classification system that separates "childhood periodic syndromes that are commonly precursors of migraines" from hemiplegic migraines, which are classified under the adult section "migraines with aura." This classification system fails to recognize that hemiplegic migraines are seen as periodic migraine precursors in children. For the sake of this chapter, the term migraine variants will be used to describe a group of stereotyped syndromes that present in children with a personal or family history of migraines. These syndromes are migraines with presenting signs and symptoms that stray from the typical and defining symptoms of classic migraine. While classic migraines are defined by throbbing focal (usually unilateral) head pain lasting one hour or more and associated with nausea, vomiting, photo- or phonophobia, and urge to sleep, migraine variants are characterized by additional symptoms that may, or may not, have cephalgia as a primary complaint.

Variants of migraines are classified by their symptoms. There are migraine variants with abdominal symptoms, which include the abdominal migraines and the cyclic vomiting syndrome. There are migraine variants that present with focal neurological deficits such as the hemiplegic migraines and the basilar migraines. Each of these subtypes will be discussed separately.

Licht DJ, Ryan NR, eds. *Curbside Consultation in Pediatric Neurology: 49 Clinical Questions* (pp 99-104).
© 2016 Taylor & Francis Group.

Migraines With Abdominal Symptoms

CYCLIC VOMITING

Cyclic vomiting is characterized by repeated, stereotyped occurrences of intense vomiting. The episodes of vomiting occur at regular intervals. In some patients, diaries reveal striking regularity of the vomiting spells. Each episode of cyclic vomiting can last hours to days and often requires hospitalization for rehydration therapy. Parents report that there are no useful interventions once the vomiting begins, and that the episodes run their course and end after a predictable/stereotyped period of time.

Initial presentations of cyclic vomiting can be quite dramatic and resemble an acute abdomen. Presentations often require a medical workup to rule out other causes of abdominal crises such as gastroenteritis, appendicitis, intestinal obstruction, or inherited metabolic disorders (Table 21-1). The first presentation of cyclic vomiting almost always occurs before the age of 10 years but is most frequent between 3 and 4 years of age. There are no gender preferences. The vomiting spells typically resolve by 10 years of age and are transformed into, or are accompanied by, more typical migraines.

ABDOMINAL MIGRAINES

Abdominal migraines are similar to cyclic vomiting, though are less severe and may be associated with other typical migraine features such as aura and other migraine prodromes (scotomas). Symptoms include nausea, vomiting, and diarrhea and can be very similar to viral gastroenteritis accompanied by a migraine-type headache.

THERAPY

The treatment of cyclic vomiting and abdominal migraines has centered on alleviating nausea and preventing dehydration. This can be accomplished with Reglan (metoclopramide), Zofran (ondansetron), and intravenous (IV) saline (normal saline for older kids, 0.5 normal saline for younger). Prophylaxis can be accomplished with most anticonvulsants used for migraine prophylaxis. Anecdotally, this author has had the most success with Neurontin (gabapentin) at doses greater than 30 mg/kg/day divided in 3 doses.

Migraines With Focal Neurological Deficits

HEMIPLEGIC MIGRAINES

Hemiplegic migraines are a group of disorders that are manifest by focal neurological deficits followed by severe migraine headache that resolve completely. The focal neurological deficits can be motor weakness, aphasia (or speech disturbance), hemianopia (loss of a visual field affecting both eyes), ataxia, or any of a myriad of symptoms that resemble acute arterial stroke.

Hemiplegic migraines can be further classified into familial or sporadic, referring to their genetics. There are 3 known genes that are associated with familial and sporadic hemiplegic migraines. In general, genetic testing has a much higher yield in familial cases (40% hit rate) than sporadic (< 10% hit rate).

Table 21-1

Symptoms and Differential Diagnosis Associated With Migraine Variants

Migraine Variant		Migraine Symptoms	Variant Symptoms	Differential Diagnosis	Age at Onset	Episode Duration	Treatment		Other
Group	Subgroup						Acute	Prophylactic	
With abdominal symptoms	Cyclic vomiting	None until age 10 years	Profuse vomiting Variable abdominal pain Occasionally altered consciousness	Intestinal obstruction Metabolic disease Raised intracranial pressure Ureto-pelvic obstruction	3 to 5 years (resolved or transformed after 10 years)	Hours to 7 days	Benzodiazepines Zofran Reglan Intravenous (IV) fluids	Gabapentin Amitriptyline Propranolol	
	Abdominal migraines	Auras, scotomas, photo-, phonophobia	Epigastric pain, mild vomiting	Peptic or gastric ulcer Cholecystitis Reflux Inflammatory bowel disease	5 to 10 years (include head pain after 10 years)	Hours to 1 day (rarely more than 1 day)	Nonsteroidal anti-inflammatory drugs Triptans Zofran	Gabapentin Cyproheptadine Valproic acid Propranolol	

(continued)

Table 21-1 (continued)

Symptoms and Differential Diagnosis Associated With Migraine Variants

Migraine Variant		Migraine Symptoms	Variant Symptoms	Differential Diagnosis	Age at Onset	Episode Duration	Treatment		Other
Group	Subgroup						Acute	Prophylactic	
With focal neurological deficits	Hemiplegic migraines	Unilateral throbbing pain Scotomas Nausea/vomiting Phono-/photophobia	Hemiplegia, contralateral to pain Hemianopia Aphasia Neglect	Stroke (must be ruled out) Tumor Mitochondrial disease	Any age, but most common in second decade (may be familial or sporadic)	Hours to days	Diamox IV Verapamil	Diamox Verapamil Flunarizine	Triptans contraindicated Genetic testing available
	Basilar migraines	Unilateral throbbing pain Scotomas Nausea/vomiting Phono-/photophobia	Dysarthria Vertigo Tinnitus Diplopia Ataxia Clouded consciousness	Stroke Transient ischemic attack Vestibular dysfunction	Any age, but most common in second decade	5 to 60 minutes with headache lasting longer	Nonsteroidal anti-inflammatory drugs Topiramate		
	Paroxysmal toricollis	None (nonspecific irritability)	Head tilt to either side	Reflux Dystonia Seizure	First year (typically 6 months)	Minutes to days (typically hours)	Cyproheptadine	Cyproheptadine	

Calcium Channel, Voltage-Dependent, P/Q Type, Alpha 1A Subunit *(CACNA1A)*

Familial hemiplegic migraine type 1 (FHM1), commonly presenting with nystagmus and other cerebellar signs, was previously estimated to account for 50% of FHM. No new studies have been conducted to improve our knowledge of the incidence. The gene is located on chromosome 19 (19p13) and codes for a voltage-sensitive calcium channel. There are at least 18 mutations that have been associated with FHM1. Some mutations are associated with hemiplegic spells that are provoked by mild head trauma. Acute magnetic resonance imaging (MRI) of the brain may be abnormal in these cases, with unilateral and focal brain edema that resolves with resolution of the migraine spell.

- *CACNA1A* is uncommonly associated with sporadic hemiplegic migraine.
- *CACNA1A* mutations are also known to cause episodic ataxia type 2 and spinocerebellar ataxia type 6.

ATPase, Na+/K+ Transporting, Alpha 2 Polypeptide *(ATP1A2)*

Familial hemiplegic migraine type 2 (FHM2), frequently occurring with epilepsy, appeared in the past to be less prevalent than FHM1, with far fewer case reports in the literature. The gene is located on chromosome 1 (1q23.2) and codes for a subunit of the sodium-potassium ATPase. More than 20 mutations have been described in both familial and sporadic cases.

- A single *ATP1A2* mutation has been described to cause a form of alternating hemiplegia of childhood (AHC).
- AHC is more commonly caused by mutations in ATPase, Na +/K + transporting, alpha 3 polypeptide (*ATP1A3*), but has also been described with glucose transporter 1 (*GLUT1*) mutations.

Sodium Channel, Voltage-Gated, Type I, Alpha Subunit *(SCN1A)*

Familial hemiplegic migraine type 3 (FHM3) has been reported in several unrelated families in the literature. Only 3 mutations in this gene, which codes for a voltage-gated sodium channel, have been described to cause FHM3. No cases of sporadic hemiplegic migraine have been associated with mutations in *SCN1A*.

- More than 150 mutations in *SCN1A* have been described in childhood seizure syndromes including generalized epilepsy with febrile seizures plus (GEFS +), Dravet syndrome, and severe myoclonic epilepsy of infancy.

Therapy

The single most important thing to remember with all hemiplegic migraine sufferers is that the use of triptans (a group of medications including sumatriptan, zolmitriptan, rizatriptan, and about 10 others) is strictly contraindicated because of the potential to convert the hemiplegic migraine into a stroke. Diamox (acetazolamide) IV or orally has been used successfully both to treat hemiplegic migraines acutely and as prophylaxis against attacks. Verapamil and other calcium channel antagonists (flunarizine) have also been proposed as specific treatments for patients with *CACNA1A* mutations but have also been used in patients with *ATP1A2* mutations as well.

Basilar Migraine

This refers to a particular subset of migraine with aura that includes vertigo, change in hearing, sleepiness, and weakness or sensory symptoms on both sides of the body.

Paroxysmal Torticollis

This very rare disorder results in a child's neck being turned and head inclined to one side. Occurring in infants and young children, this migraine variant can also be accompanied by nausea and vomiting. Episodes may last from a few hours to a few days. Cephalgia may be manifested by irritability during the spell.

Confusional Migraine

Some children do have more dramatic auras that can include change in level of consciousness, confusion, and even bizarre visual illusions and spatial distortions associated with their migraine headache (ie, "Alice in Wonderland" syndrome). These symptoms can be prolonged, lasting for many hours. Cephalgia may coexist with the confusion or arrive with the clearing of mental status. To ensure no more serious underlying cause can be found, any child with a headache and the above symptoms should be evaluated by a physician.

Suggested Readings

International Headache Society. *The International Headache Classification.* 2nd ed. http://ihs-classification.org/en/

Lateef T, Cui L, Heaton L, et al. Validation of a migraine interview for children and adolescents. *Pediatrics.* 2013;131(1):e96-e102.

Lewis D, Ashwal S, Hershey A, Hirtz D, Yonker M, Silberstein S. Practice parameter: pharmacological treatment of migraine headache in children and adolescents: report of the American Academy of Neurology Quality Standards Subcommittee and the Practice Committee of the Child Neurology Society. *Neurology.* 2004;63(12):2215-2224.

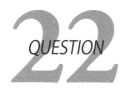

WHAT CAN BE DONE FOR A POST-CONCUSSIVE HEADACHE?

Nicole R. Ryan, MD

Owing to the increasing knowledge of the negative long-term cognitive outcomes in adults and children with multiple concussions, head injury has recently taken a spotlight in the media. Most states have now adopted laws that require a child with a sports-related concussion to be evaluated by a trained medical professional prior to returning to play. This has significantly increased the number of children with concussion presenting for medical care and forced primary physicians as well as specialists to obtain skills in concussion management.

While many symptoms are reported following a concussion, the most common and at times disabling complaint is headache. These headaches are typically migraine or tension-type headaches and are associated with photophobia, phonophobia, and nausea. Many patients may present to the pediatrician wearing sunglasses because of light sensitivity. While concussion can lead to cognitive impairments irrespective of headache, often the headache can further exacerbate the inability to concentrate, and concentration will usually worsen pain. Headache can also lead to difficulty falling asleep, another common post-concussive complaint. It is important to obtain a detailed history of other symptoms including poor concentration, sleep, dizziness, and mood disturbance to determine how these might be contributing to headache symptoms.

The acute and chronic management of post-concussive headache differs. Acutely, patients should be placed both on physical and cognitive rest.[1] Children who are pushed back to school and activities immediately tend to have longer recovery times. Approaches to medical management of headache early do differ and there are no guidelines for treatment of post-concussive headache. Our practice is to discourage nonsteroidal anti-inflammatory use unless it is necessary to help a child sleep. This is both to prevent rebound headache from overuse but also to prevent a child from engaging in overactivity due to masked symptoms, possibly prolonging headache. Should the headache worsen, rest and hydration are the initial mainstays of treatment. Most patients will recover within 1 to 4 weeks using these strategies alone.

Licht DJ, Ryan NR, eds. *Curbside Consultation in Pediatric Neurology: 49 Clinical Questions* (pp 105-106). © 2016 Taylor & Francis Group.

As discussed in Question 30, the length of recovery that defines "post-concussive syndrome" is controversial and often longer in children. If post-concussive headache continues beyond 4 to 6 weeks, the phase of acute injury is over, and I have found that a staged return to activities irrespective of symptoms improves overall recovery. In order to start "pushing" a child back to school and exercise, pain must be addressed often using a multimodal approach.

First, lifestyle changes must be addressed. Often, particularly if the child has not attended school for several weeks, sleep is disordered, and he or she is going to bed late and waking late. Gradually altering this schedule to one similar to a school day often helps not only school return but also headache. I discourage napping more than 15 to 20 minutes at a time although short rest breaks during the day are an important part of recovery and should be part of a return to school plan. Hydration must again be emphasized. Exercise at gradually increasing intervals and intensity must be initiated. This is also the stage at which therapies, particularly vestibular or occupational therapies for eye movement abnormalities that can contribute to headache and/or physical therapy for aerobic activity, can be initiated. In some areas, there are brain injury/concussion rehabilitation programs that include these services to which a patient can be referred. To address the stress of a prolonged injury, relaxation and breathing techniques can be tried as well as massage or acupuncture. Often muscular neck tension is present in post-concussive patients that exacerbates headache symptoms, and I have even found botulinum toxin or nerve blocks to be effective in refractory post-concussive headaches. Biofeedback is a known treatment for chronic migraine and can also be effective in post-concussive patients.

As post-concussive headaches are typically migraine or chronic tension-type headaches, prophylactic medications can be helpful in this group. As sleep disturbance tends to also be a comorbid symptom, amitriptyline or nortriptyline are often good first-line choices for prophylactic medications. Although there is one study of blast injury in military personnel suggesting topiramate may be superior to amitriptyline in post-concussive headache,[2] topiramate is often avoided owing to concerns of worsening cognitive deficits. I have also used cyproheptadine (also with benefits for sleep), gabapentin, and verapamil with some success for post-concussive headache.

Overall, while most post-concussive headaches resolve in the acute period, headaches associated with post-concussive syndrome can be refractory to treatment and most of the evidence for response is anecdotal. A multimodal treatment approach, emphasizing lifestyle changes, therapies, and medications, often produces the best results. Maintaining a positive outlook for recovery when talking to your patients can also make a significant difference as psychosocial factors almost invariably play a role in patients with prolonged symptoms.

References

1. Moser R, Glatts C, Schatz P. Efficacy of immediate and delayed cognitive and physical rest for treatment of sports-related concussion. *J Pediatr.* 2012;161:922-926.
2. Erickson JC. Treatment outcome of chronic posttraumatic headaches after mild trauma in US soldiers: an observational study. *Headache.* 2011;51:932-944.

SECTION IV

FLOPPY BABY

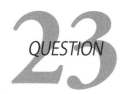

WHAT ARE THE MOST IMPORTANT COMPONENTS OF THE EXAM IN EVALUATING A HYPOTONIC BABY?

Sabrina W. Yum, MD

Evaluation of Muscle Tone

Muscle tone and power should be evaluated when the child is awake and comfortable and should be delayed, if possible, in sick children or children with malnutrition. The evaluation can also be compromised by medications. Muscle tone is divided into 2 types: appendicular tone (muscle tone in the limbs) and axial tone (truncal tone). It is important to distinguish hypotonia (reduced resistance to passive range of motion) from muscle weakness (reduced maximum power generated). A weak infant is often hypotonic whereas a hypotonic infant need not be weak.

All hypotonic infants look similar when lying supine with a "frog leg" posture and paucity of spontaneous movement. Poor head control and head lag are seen on "pull to sit." There is slip through on vertical suspension, and an inverted U posture on horizontal suspension (Landau maneuver). With stimulation, the hypotonic infants without muscle weakness may demonstrate antigravity limb movements. Other signs of weakness include weak cry, paradoxical breathing pattern (belly breathing), swallowing difficulty manifesting as slow feeding, oropharyngeal pooling of secretion or food, or choking.

History, Clinical Clues on Examination, and Diagnostic Approach

Hypotonia is seen in diseases affecting the brain and spinal cord (central nervous system [CNS]) or diseases of the anterior horn cells, peripheral nerves, neuromuscular junction, and

Licht DJ, Ryan NR, eds. *Curbside Consultation in Pediatric Neurology: 49 Clinical Questions* (pp 109-113).

Table 23-1
Differential Diagnosis of Infantile Hypotonia

Central Hypotonia (With Upper Motor Neuron Signs)
- Brain or spinal cord: hypoxic ischemic injury, trauma, infection, malformations
- Metabolic and endocrine etiology: hypothyroidism, Zellweger syndrome, neonatal adrenoleukodystrophy, biotinidase deficiency, mitochondrial diseases, aminoacidopathies, organic acidurias, urea cycle disorders and others
- Chromosomal: trisomy 21, Prader-Willi syndrome and others

Peripheral Hypotonia (With Lower Motor Neuron Signs)
- Anterior horn cell disease: spinal muscular atrophy, infantile neuroaxonal dystrophy, poliomyelitis
- Peripheral neuropathy: Charcot-Marie-Tooth disease, chronic inflammatory demyelinating neuropathy, Guillain-Barré syndrome
- Neuromuscular junction defect: transitory myasthenia gravis, congenital myasthenic syndrome, infant botulism
- Muscle:
  - Muscular dystrophy: congenital myotonic dystrophy, congenital muscular dystrophy
  - Metabolic myopathies: glycogen-storage disease type II (Pompe), mitochondrial cytopathy
  - Congenital myopathy: nemaline myopathy, myotubular myopathy, central nuclear myopathy, central core myopathy, congenital fiber type disproportion and others
  - Infantile myositis
- Connective tissue: collagen VI disease (Ullrich muscular dystrophy)

muscles (peripheral nervous system [PNS]). Distinctive features in birth and medical history, family history, or physical examination frequently allow localization of the lesion to the CNS or PNS, or both. Patients with peripheral hypotonia often have depressed deep tendon reflexes, but this feature is not helpful in separating neuropathies from myopathies. The localization of the disease will help to quickly narrow the list of differential diagnoses (Table 23-1) and guide subsequent investigations. The incidence of decreased fetal movements, polyhydramnios, or breech presentation is higher in fetuses with neuromuscular disorders. A history of delivery complications, anoxia/hypoxia, low cord pH and Apgar scores, seizures, or syndromic features (facial dysmorphisms or other congenital malformations) offers support for a central origin. Many patients with central hypotonia may evolve to have appendicular hypertonia while retaining axial hypotonia. Other useful clinical clues for central vs peripheral hypotonia are listed in Table 23-2.

Table 23-2
Clinical Clues of Central and Peripheral Hypotonia

Clinical Features	Central Hypotonia	Peripheral Hypotonia
Other abnormal brain function (such as impaired mental status, seizure, cognitive impairment, microcephaly)	++	− (Except in some forms of congenital muscular dystrophy, myotonic dystrophy)
Malformation of other organs	±	−
Dysmorphic features	±	−
Tendon reflexes	Brisk or normal	Depressed or absent
Postural reflexes	Preserved	Depressed or absent
Fisting of hands	+	−
Scissoring of legs	±	−
Atrophy of muscles	−	+
Limb weakness	±	+++
Facial weakness	−	Variable
Fasciculation of tongue	−	+ In spinal muscular atrophy

Diagnostic Testing

Diagnostic testing should be guided by clinical findings and performed in a stepwise manner. There are usually sufficient clinical findings that allow the selection of only a few diagnostic tests as a priority, and in some cases, specific clinical signs may emerge with longer follow-up.

Special investigations should be delayed in those with acute systemic illness and malnutrition if possible, as reversible hypotonia and weakness are frequently seen in these settings. Neonatal hypotonia, hyporeflexia, and respiratory depression can be associated with hypermagnesemia due to magnesium sulfate infusion to the mother with eclampsia. The finding of thrombocytosis and abnormal liver function should raise concern for in utero infection and prompt further investigation with TORCH titers, particularly in neonates with microcephaly, in utero growth retardation, and hearing impairment. Serum albumin, calcium, phosphorus, alkaline phosphatase level, and thyroid function will provide confirmation for malnutrition, rickets, and hypothyroidism.

For patients with central hypotonia, a brain magnetic resonance imaging can confirm hypoxic ischemic encephalopathy, brain malformation, neuronal migration defect, and white matter diseases. Genome-wide microarray has proven to be a powerful tool for the detection of submicroscopic chromosomal abnormalities, especially in those with dysmorphic features.

The majority of neuromuscular diseases in infants and young children are genetic conditions. Special diagnostic testing can be performed to further localize the lesion in the motor units, which can guide further genetic testing for confirmation of diagnosis. The normal newborn may have elevated serum creatine kinase (CK) during the first few days after birth and neonates with

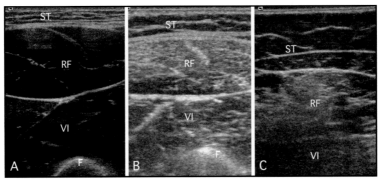

Figure 23-1. Axial muscle ultrasound of the mid-thigh of (A) a healthy 9-year-old boy, (B) a 5-year-old girl with congenital muscular dystrophy, and (C) a 5-year-old boy with spinal muscular atrophy type III. In healthy individuals, muscles appear (A) largely black with few perimysial septa. In the myopathic condition, muscles show (B) increased homogeneous granular echogenicity. In the neurogenic condition, muscles typically show (C) streak-like, inhomogeneous echogenicity, and fasciculation can be observed in many cases of neurogenic diseases (not shown). RF: rectus femoris; VI: vastus intermedius; ST: subcutaneous tissue; F: femur.

asphyxia may have CK as high as 1000 IU/L, but the level should be normalized with time. Markedly elevated CK (> 10× normal) is frequently seen in muscular dystrophies and inflammatory myopathy, as well as certain metabolic myopathies, but a normal serum CK level is typically seen in patients with congenital myopathies or collagen diseases. Serum CK level may be normal to moderately elevated (up to 5 times normal) in spinal muscular atrophy.

Nerve conduction and electromyography help to differentiate neurogenic from myopathic process, and is essential in classifying neuropathy as axonal or demyelinating. The study can be technically challenging in neonates and young children and should be performed only by experienced physicians.

Muscles ultrasound is a very useful, noninvasive technique for visualizing normal and pathological skeletal muscle. It can be performed at bedside without sedation but requires significant training for interpretation. In neuromuscular diseases, an increase in fatty tissues, fibrosis, and inflammation result in increased muscle echogenicity. The appearance of echogenicity and the pattern of muscle involvement can guide localization or differential diagnosis (Figure 23-1).

Muscle biopsy with histology, specific staining techniques, and electron microscopy is essential for morphologic diagnosis and remains helpful in diagnosing specific forms of congenital myopathies even with the recent advance of genetic testing. Nerve biopsy is rarely helpful in diagnosing Charcot-Marie-Tooth disease but may be performed on occasion when chronic inflammatory demyelinating neuropathy is suspected, especially in patients with atypical features and poor response to standard therapies.

Genetic testing should be guided by clinical evaluation, and targeted studies are preferred. The availability of next-generation sequencing (high-throughput sequencing technologies that parallelize the sequencing process, producing thousands or millions of sequences concurrently) and whole exome sequencing (selectively sequencing the coding regions of the genome) have allowed identification of gene mutations that cause many undiagnosed childhood neuromuscular and neurological diseases. However, it has added much more complexity and raised ethical issues. There is growing concern that complete sequencing data lead to weakly justified claims of association between genetic variants and disease. Proper genetic counseling must be provided before and after the testing, and the ordering physicians should be prepared to interpret the results, especially variants that have not been reported (or variants of unknown clinical significance) and to address unexpected and unrelated findings.

In infants with hepatosplenomegaly and cardiomyopathy on exam, Pompe disease, a glycogen-storage disease with available enzyme replacement treatment, should be considered, and can be diagnosed with enzymatic analysis and confirmed by genetic testing.

Principles of Management

It is important to recognize treatable conditions so specific therapies can be administered in a timely manner to minimize permanent damage/long-term neurological sequelae. Babies with hypotonia caused by an infection, electrolyte disturbances, and hypothyroidism will usually improve with successful treatment of the underlying condition.

Feeding problems are frequently encountered in patients with hypotonia, especially those with peripheral hypotonia due to oral pharyngeal muscle weakness. Special nipples, small and frequent feeding, gavage feeding, or even gastrostomy tube feeding may be needed. The risk for aspiration pneumonia should be assessed. Frequent suctioning, postural drainage, and a vigorous respiratory therapy regimen are required in patients with impaired cough reflex and bulbar weakness. Hypoventilation and hypercapnia need to be evaluated and managed by pulmonary specialists. Progressive scoliosis, and a rigid spine and chest wall may further compromise respiratory status and should be monitored closely and managed by orthopedics.

Some metabolic diseases are treatable. Many types of aminoacidopathies, organic acidurias, and urea cycle disorders can be treated with special diet and vitamins, and in the emergency setting, detoxification methods such as dialysis may be considered. Enzyme-replacement therapy such as Myozyme (alglucosidase alfa) has changed the clinical course of infantile form of Pompe disease. Some lysosomal disorders can be efficiently treated by enzyme-replacement or substrate-reduction therapies.

Physical and occupational therapy remain the mainstays of therapy for most patients. It is essential that families be educated on the importance of a daily home exercise/stretch program. The objectives are to prevent contracture, maintain range of motion, and promote motor learning and independence. Well-fitted orthotics can be quite helpful. Some patients with severe contractures may need tendon-release or lengthening surgery.

Suggested Readings

Engel AG. Current status of the congenital myasthenic syndromes. *Neuromuscular Disorders*. 2012;22:99-111.

North KN, Wang CH, Clarke N, et al. Approach to the diagnosis of congenital myopathies. *Neuromuscular Disorders*. 2014;24:97-116.

Schoser B, Hill V, Raben N. Therapeutic approaches in glycogen storage disease type II (GSDII)/Pompe disease *Neurotherapeutics*. 2008;5:569-578. doi:10.1016/j.nurt.2008.08.009

Wang CH, Bonnemann CG, Rutkowski A, et al. Consensus statement on standard of care for congenital muscular dystrophies. *J Child Neurol*. 2010;25:1559-1581.

Wang CH, Finkel RS, Bertini ES, et al. Consensus statement for standard of care in spinal muscular atrophy. *J Child Neurol*. 2007;22:1027-1049.

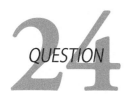

HOW DO I DISTINGUISH CENTRAL FROM PERIPHERAL CAUSES OF HYPOTONIA?

Michele L. Yang, MD

One of the most common diagnostic challenges a pediatric clinician faces is the hypotonic child. The sheer number of potential diagnoses can initially appear overwhelming. Hypotonia can result from dysfunction anywhere along the neuroaxis, including the brain, spinal cord, nerve, neuromuscular junction, and muscle, as well as from genetic and metabolic causes. Identifying an etiology is important for discussions about prognosis, management strategies, anticipatory care, and assessment of accurate recurrence risks for future children. A simple approach to this problem is to distinguish between central and peripheral causes of hypotonia.[1,2] A detailed history and careful examination are the only tools needed initially. Table 24-1 outlines the common clues that distinguish between central and peripheral hypotonia. Once this distinction has been made, determining tiered testing for central and peripheral causes becomes much less daunting. This simplified approach is as follows.

Defining Hypotonia

Before starting an evaluation, the clinician must understand the definition of hypotonia. A child can appear floppy either because of decreased tone or because of weakness, and therefore a distinction should be made between the 2. Tone is the resistance of muscles to passive movement around a joint. Therefore, hypotonia is the decreased resistance of muscle to passive movement around a joint. Weakness is due to decreased muscle power or strength generated by active movement. While weak children are always hypotonic, hypotonic children may have normal strength.

Licht DJ, Ryan NR, eds. *Curbside Consultation in Pediatric Neurology: 49 Clinical Questions* (pp 115-118).
© 2016 Taylor & Francis Group.

Table 24-1

Common Clinical Clues for
Central vs Peripheral Causes of Hypotonia

Central Hypotonia	*Peripheral Hypotonia*
• Dysmorphic features • Cognitive and language delays • Normal strength • Increased reflexes • Clonus • Crossed adductors • Seizures • Fisting of hands • Depressed level of consciousness • Predominantly axial hypotonia and weakness	• Muscle fasciculations • Weakness, such as lack of antigravity movements or lack of spontaneous movements • Depressed or absent reflexes • Normal cognitive and language function • Limited eye movements • Decreased muscle bulk or muscle atrophy • Myopathic facies: long, narrow facies with tented upper lip

Obtaining a Detailed History

The history is a crucial part of the evaluation. For an infant with hypotonia, the birth history can help estimate the onset of symptoms. Lack of fetal movements throughout the pregnancy, indicating a prenatal onset, is commonly seen in patients with the congenital muscular dystrophies and myopathies. Infants who are born with normal movements and tone who become hypotonic after 24 to 48 hours may have a metabolic disorder. A history of maternal exposures or infections can suggest a central nervous system (CNS) etiology, as can an abnormal fetal ultrasound of the brain. Amniotic fluid volume is important to note, as children with bulbar weakness may have a history of oligohydramnios or polyhydramnios. The delivery history can equally provide clues. The mode of delivery, complications encountered during delivery, evidence of asphyxia, and Apgar scores can be telling regarding the etiology. Asphyxia and low Apgar scores are common presentations for hypoxic-ischemic encephalopathy, one of the most common causes of neonatal hypotonia. A family history of seizures, cognitive delay, and malformations suggests a search for CNS etiologies. On the other hand, a family history of muscle cramping, exercise intolerance, weakness, and early loss of ambulation may suggest a neuromuscular etiology. The child's developmental history is important to assess whether decreased tone occurs in the context of language and cognitive delays, which would suggest a CNS etiology. A progressive loss of skills suggests a neurodegenerative disorder. The longitudinal course can also provide clues about the etiology. For instance, cervical cord trauma can present with neonatal hypotonia, with other neurological signs and manifesting days to weeks later. A detailed review of systems is essential to determine the presence of other associated systemic involvement. A history of current or past seizures would suggest CNS etiologies. Liver failure or intolerance of feeds can be seen in metabolic disorders.

Performing a Focused Examination

The key to the examination of the child is watchful observation in order to localize central or peripheral dysfunction. More information can be gleaned from observation of a child than auscultation, palpation, and percussion in a formal examination. In certain age groups, the direct approach of starting the examination with the head and finishing with the feet is doomed to failure. Many crucial aspects of the examination can be noted simply by watching the child in a quiet, alert state. For example, a hypotonic infant in supine lies with abducted hips and knees flexed, in a "frog-legged" position. A lack of spontaneous movements suggests weakness. Observing normal feeding and playing provides information about bulbar function and facial movements, and muscle strength, respectively. In an ambulatory child, observation of gait, stair climb, and the degree of difficulty arising from the ground are excellent methods of detecting proximal weakness. Dysmorphic features should be noted, as they can suggest a genetic or metabolic syndrome. A long, narrow face with limited facial expression is often associated with muscle weakness. Particular attention should be paid to abnormal hair, teeth, skin, and nails, because they, like the brain, are of neuroectodermal origin and may reflect CNS lesions. Once the child begins to warm up to the examiner, mental status, including assessment of language, can be performed through interactive play. A child with a dull appearance or encephalopathy likely has CNS involvement as a cause of hypotonia.

After a period of observation, the formal examination should be performed with particular attention to testing tone, assessing muscle strength, and obtaining reflexes. Extremity tone is assessed by passive movements of the arms and legs. Truncal and nuchal tone are assessed by performing horizontal suspension, vertical suspension, and traction response. In horizontal suspension, the infant is suspended in prone with the examiner's hand under the chest. The hypotonic infant's head and limbs hang limply, forming an inverted U shape. In vertical suspension, the examiner holds the infant with both hands under the arms. The hypotonic infant "slips through" at the shoulders when this maneuver is performed. For the traction response, the infant lies in supine on the exam table and is pulled into a sitting position by the arms. Head lag is present when this is performed in a hypotonic infant.

In distinguishing between a peripheral and central cause of hypotonia, the deep tendon reflexes are likely the most valuable part of the examination. Brisk reflexes and clonus indicate CNS dysfunction. Decreased or absent reflexes indicate a disorder of the lower motor neuron or muscle.

Formal testing of muscle strength in children can be challenging, and therefore, the muscle strength evaluation often relies on observation during the first part of the visit. In older children, grading muscle strength can be performed on a 5-point scale. Accurate assessment of muscle strength, however, should be made based on age-appropriate norms.

Examination of the parents should be considered an extension of the examination of the child. In particular, if neuromuscular disorders are being considered, the parents should be examined. For example, in patients with congenital myotonic dystrophy, one of the parents, most often the mother, will have grip myotonia when shaking hands. These parents may not report symptoms; therefore, unless an effort is made to examine the parents, important clues may be overlooked.

Once a central or peripheral cause has been determined, screening investigations can be initiated (Table 24-2). As a general rule, whenever motor delay or hypotonia is present, a serum creatine kinase (CK) should be obtained. Remember: "If there is delay, check a CK." This simple test can help identify neuromuscular involvement and initiate workup for muscle disease. While genetic technology has become increasingly sophisticated, allowing us to identify novel genes, studies have shown that with history and examination alone, a successful diagnosis can be made in 63% of children with hypotonia.[1] In short, the decades-old problem of a hypotonic child is still approached using the simplest of tools: the history and the examination.

Table 24-2

Investigations for Causes of Central vs Peripheral Hypotonia

	Central Hypotonia	*Peripheral Hypotonia*
Tier 1	MRI brain Chromosomal microarray	Creatine kinase Lactate Pyruvate Consider SMN testing or DMPK (if spinal muscular atrophy or myotonic dystrophy suspected)
Tier 2	Lactate/pyruvate Serum electrolytes, thyroid function tests If metabolic disorders considered, check serum amino acids and urine organic acids	MRI brain: to evaluate if associated CNS abnormalities are present, as can be seen with congenital muscular dystrophies
Tier 3	Plasma cooper/ceruloplasmin assay Very long chain fatty acids Ophthalmologic evaluation	EMG/NCS Muscle biopsy

MRI: magnetic resonance imaging; SMN: survival motor neuron; DMPK: dystrophia myotonica-protein kinase; CNS: central nervous system; EMG: electromyogram; NCS: nerve conduction studies.

References

1. Paro-Panjan F, Neubauer D. Congenital hypotonia: is there an algorithm? *J Child Neurol.* 2004;19(6):439-442.
2. Laugel V, Cossée M, Matis J, et al. Diagnostic approach to neonatal hypotonia. *Eur J Pediatr.* 2008;167(5):517-523.

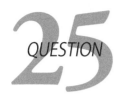

WHAT ARE THE MOST COMMON GENETIC CAUSES OF HYPOTONIA?

Michele L. Yang, MD

Genetic disorders should be suspected in infants with central hypotonia with dysmorphic features, abnormal head circumference, growth abnormalities, and global developmental delay with cognitive defects. Of the genetic disorders causing central hypotonia, Down syndrome is one of the most common causes. It can often be identified clinically by the characteristic facies seen in children with trisomy 21, including upward slanting palpebral fissures, epicanthal folds, midface hypoplasia, and a single transverse palmar crease. Simple karyotype testing provides genetic confirmation and rules out other forms of aneuploidy (abnormal number of chromosomes). Another common genetic disorder presenting with hypotonia is Prader-Willi syndrome, which often presents in infancy with severe hypotonia, poor feeding, and hypogonadism/hypoplastic genitalia. At about 1 year of age, these children typically are of short stature and develop hyperphagia with rapid weight gain. In later childhood, they have some degree of cognitive impairment, hypothalamic hypogonadism, and behavioral problems. The mainstay of diagnosis is DNA methylation testing to detect abnormal parent-specific imprinting within chromosome 15q11-13.[1] This testing detects more than 99% of affected individuals. Genome-wide single-nucleotide polymorphism (SNP) array will also uncover "uniparental disomy" (both alleles coming from one parent) at 15q11-13.

Another relatively common cause of peripheral hypotonia in the infant is myotonic dystrophy. Neonates with congenital myotonic dystrophy are typically born to affected mothers. To the experienced provider, the diagnosis can be made when meeting the parents, even before seeing the infant. A mother with myotonic dystrophy will have characteristic facies (high forehead, temporal wasting, ptosis, and/or drooping of the lips) and trouble letting go after shaking hands, a sign of myotonia. The affected neonate often has a difficult peri- and postnatal course. The labor can be prolonged, requiring mechanical assistance. At birth, these infants have significant hypotonia, bifacial weakness, and proximal weakness. They may require mechanical ventilation owing to respiratory muscle weakness, and nutritional support because of oromotor dysfunction. Respiratory

Licht DJ, Ryan NR, eds. *Curbside Consultation in
Pediatric Neurology: 49 Clinical Questions* (pp 119-121).
© 2016 Taylor & Francis Group.

failure and an increased risk of aspiration can lead to early death. If the infant survives past the first 3 postnatal weeks, motor function may improve, though bifacial weakness typically persists. Cognitive deficits can be profound in patients with congenital myotonic dystrophy. This neuromuscular disorder results from an expansion of cytosine-thymine-guanine repeats on chromosome 19. Anticipation with increased repeats occurs when the disorder is inherited maternally, with successive generations being more severely affected. It is therefore essential that the parents be examined for signs of weakness and myotonia when considering this diagnosis in a newborn.

Congenital brain malformations travel with genetic diagnoses and may also result in central hypotonia in infancy. Increasingly, genetic causes of brain malformations are being identified. For instance, classic Joubert syndrome is characterized by distinctive cerebellar and brainstem malformations, hypotonia, and developmental delays. The classic clinical and imaging findings may prompt a workup. At this time, 18 genes are known to be associated with this constellation of signs. X-linked lissencephaly is caused by a mutation in the aristaless-related homeobox (*ARX*) or doublecortin (*DCX*) gene, and is seen primarily in males, though females may be affected with brain malformations, seizures, and some degree of intellectual disability. Identifying the genetic causes may be helpful when providing genetic counseling for the families.

Of the peripheral disorders causing hypotonia, spinal muscular atrophy is one of the more common genetic neuromuscular disorders encountered. Spinal muscular atrophy type 1 is an autosomal recessive disorder resulting in marked, progressive weakness and hypotonia in infancy. These infants typically have a bright alert look despite their significant proximal weakness. Importantly, reflexes are absent. They may initially have varying degrees of difficulty with feeding and with respiratory muscle weakness. With progression of the disease, infants with this disorder develop respiratory failure, with most dying by their second year of life. However, increasing evidence suggests that with improved respiratory and nutritional support, life expectancy may be improved.[2] Genetic testing for deletions of exon 7 in the survival motor neuron (*SMN*, chromosome 5q13) gene confirms the diagnosis in the majority of patients.

While metabolic disorders are uncommon and rarely present with hypotonia as the sole feature, they are included here for completeness so the provider does not neglect to consider these disorders in the correct clinical context. Usually they are accompanied by dysmorphic features, multisystem organ involvement, encephalopathy, and/or seizures. For instance, the finding of an enlarged heart, macroglossia, and respiratory difficulty in a floppy, weak infant should prompt a workup for glycogen-storage disorder type II or Pompe disease.

Being able to recognize these few common genetic disorders is essential in the evaluation of the hypotonic infant (Table 25-1). In a retrospective review of hypotonic infants, in cases where a definitive diagnosis was made, 40% were made on purely clinical grounds.[3] This underscores the importance of familiarity with these causes of hypotonia.

Table 25-1

Summary of the Most Common Genetic Causes of Hypotonia

Central Hypotonia

- Genetic disorders
  - Down syndrome
  - Prader-Willi syndrome
  - Other chromosomal abnormalities
- Brain malformation
  - Agenesis of the corpus callosum
  - Dandy-Walker malformation
  - Joubert syndrome
  - Lissencephaly
- Metabolic/endocrine disorders
  - Pompe disease
  - Respiratory chain defect disorders
  - Peroxisomal disorders
  - Nonketotic hyperglycinemia
  - Methemoglobinemia
  - Hypothyroidism

Peripheral Hypotonia

- Motor neuron disease
  - Spinal muscular atrophy
- Muscle disease
  - Congenital myotonic dystrophy

References

1. Gunay-Aygun M, Schwartz S, Heeger S, O'Riordan MA, Cassidy SB. The changing purpose of Prader-Willi syndrome: clinical diagnostic criteria and proposed revised criteria. *Pediatrics.* 2001;108(5):e92.
2. Oskoui M, Levy G, Garland CJ, et al. The changing natural history of spinal muscular atrophy type 1. *Neurology.* 2007;69(20):1931-1936.
3. Birdi K, Prasad AN, Prasad C, Chodirker B, Chudley AE. The floppy infant: retrospective analysis of clinical experience (1990-2000) in a tertiary care facility. *J Child Neurol.* 2005;20(10):803-808.

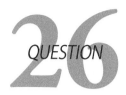

WHAT ARE THE CLINICAL FEATURES OF INFANT BOTULISM? HOW IS IT TREATED?

Jennifer L. McGuire, MD, MSCE

Infant botulism is a rare but life-threatening acute to subacute neuroparalytic disorder. It is caused by a toxin produced by the gram-positive, anaerobic, spore-forming organism *Clostridium botulinum*, found in soil, marine animals, and bird intestines. Infant botulism was first described in the United States in 1976,[1-3] and is now the most common form of botulism in the United States, causing 70 to 110 cases annually,[4,5] or 2.1 cases per 100,000 live births.[1] Infant botulism may occur in boys or girls of all ethnic groups between the ages of 2 weeks and 1 year. The median age of diagnosis is 10 to 14 weeks,[1,3] and 95% of cases occur before 6 months.[6]

Most cases of infant botulism in the United States follow the density and geography of *C botulinum* endemic in soil. Spores of identical toxin type to known cases have been found in yard soil and vacuum cleaner dust near affected infants. Farming or new construction probably disrupts the soil and wind then transmits *C botulinum* in dust particles to the infant.[4] *C botulinum* is particularly prevalent in certain regions of California, Utah, and Eastern Pennsylvania, but has been reported in at least 23 of 50 states.[2] Most children do not have a clear clinical exposure, other than recent home renovation, construction, or a parent regularly exposed to soil. Spores may also be found in honey or home-canned goods, although this is a less important source of infection in the United States (less than 20% of cases). Other risk factors for disease identified in epidemiologic studies include White race, 2-parent middle-income families, and families with older siblings. The reason for these associations is unclear, but it is possible that an as-yet-unidentified risk factor is more prevalent in these demographic groups. Other risk factors may include recent changes in diet, such as weaning from breast-feeding or introducing new food sources that change the gastrointestinal microbiological milieu.[6,7]

Upon ingestion, *C botulinum* spores move through the gastrointestinal tract to the colon, where they germinate in that anaerobic environment, and begin to produce toxin, which is absorbed by the infant.[6] Young infants are particularly vulnerable to this pathophysiology

Licht DJ, Ryan NR, eds. *Curbside Consultation in Pediatric Neurology: 49 Clinical Questions* (pp 123-126).
© 2016 Taylor & Francis Group.

because their immature intestinal flora and lack of *Clostridium*-inhibiting bile acids make their gut more susceptible to extensive colonization and toxin production.[2] Once absorbed into the bloodstream, the toxin irreversibly blocks acetylcholine release at all peripheral cholinergic junctions (motor and autonomic), resulting in failed action potentials and clinical motor and autonomic dysfunction.[5,6]

Following an incubation period of 3 to 30 days, the clinical presentation of infant botulism may vary, ranging from feeding difficulties to sudden death from respiratory arrest.[1,6] Most infants, however, initially present with constipation and poor feeding,[2] followed by a symmetric acute/subacute descending flaccid paralysis that begins with the cranial nerves (ophthalmoparesis, ptosis, poor gag, poor cough, difficulty swallowing) and descends to the upper extremities and respiratory muscles. Autonomic symptoms may include decreased tearing and salivation, a widely fluctuant heart rate and blood pressure, and flushed skin.[7] Notably, level of consciousness is normal because the toxin does not cross the blood-brain barrier. Ultimately, 50% to 70% of untreated infants will progress to respiratory failure requiring intubation and mechanical ventilation.[6] Without treatment, infants may take up to 3 months to fully clear *C botulinum* spore colonization, and even longer to fully recover peripheral cholinergic junction functionality.

The diagnosis of infant botulism is clinical and requires a high index of suspicion.[6,7] Botulism should be suspected in any previously healthy and robust infant with new head lag, cranial nerve dysfunction, inactivity, and constipation. Sepsis, the most common admission diagnosis for these children, should be ruled out in all affected infants with a complete blood count, blood and urine cultures, and lumbar puncture. A differential diagnosis of acquired acute flaccid paralysis is included in Table 26-1. Metabolic disorders and spinal muscular atrophy type 1 in particular are common mimics. In the setting of infant botulism, blood, urine, and cerebrospinal analysis/culture, metabolic, and hepatic profiles are typically normal. Electroencephalography and neuroimaging are also normal as long as there has been no hypoxic-ischemic insult from consequent respiratory failure.[3,7]

The gold standard in the diagnosis of infant botulism is the isolation of *C botulinum* spores and toxin from stool using a toxin neutralization mouse bioassay and polymerase chain reaction performed at a state lab or by the Centers for Disease Control and Prevention.[7] However, stool collection may be difficult because of constipation, and toxin assays and cultures may take up to 6 days to produce results, leading to a significant delay to treatment if all cases were confirmed.[3] Serum samples are specific but not sensitive. Electrophysiologic testing classically demonstrates an abnormal electroincremental response to rapid repetitive stimulation and short-duration, low-amplitude motor unit potentials. However, these findings are not pathognomonic of infant botulism and will be found only in affected muscle groups later in the course of disease, so a normal study does not necessarily rule out the diagnosis.

All infants with a clinical diagnosis of infant botulism should be empirically treated with botulinum immune globulin for infants (babyBIG) while awaiting confirmatory testing. BabyBIG is derived from pooled plasma of immunized adult volunteers, and serves to neutralize free toxin.[4] It is obtained by contacting the California Department of Health Services (www.infantbotulism.org), having a brief physician-to-physician discussion, filling out minimal paperwork, and receiving approval from the hospital's institutional financial officer. BabyBIG is then express-shipped to the child and given as a single dose of 50 mg/kg[4]; its long half-life neutralizes toxin for at least 6 months thereafter.[7] Prompt babyBIG administration within 3 days of admission has been shown to reduce average length of hospital stay by 3.1 weeks, length of intensive care unit admission by 3.2 weeks, duration of mechanical ventilation by 2.6 weeks, and duration of mechanical feeding by 6.4 weeks. This corresponds to a gross savings of $88,600 per patient.[5] Management of affected infants is otherwise supportive, including maintaining the infant supine with head of the bed at 30 degrees to minimize risk for aspiration, maintaining a roll behind their necks and thighs to minimize venous pooling,

Table 26-1
Differential Diagnosis of Acute/Subacute Flaccid Paralysis in Infants

Diagnosis	*Distinguishing Features*
Guillain-Barré syndrome	Typically an *ascending* flaccid paralysis in older children, with prominent sensory changes. Presentation does not include constipation.
Myasthenia gravis	Symptoms fluctuate and worsen with exertion. Presentation does not include mydriasis or constipation.
Spinal muscular atrophy type I (Werdnig-Hoffmann disease)	Symptoms present subacutely or indolently and are progressive. Typical presentation is with gross motor milestone delay. Early ptosis, mydriasis, ophthalmoplegia, and constipation are not common features.
Metabolic disorders	Electrolyte abnormalities, hypothyroidism, hepatic encephalopathy, mitochondrial and peroxisomal disorders, amino and organic acidemias may be diagnosed with blood work.
Toxins	Alcohol, narcotics, heavy metal poisoning, organophosphates, and anticholinergic ingestion should be considered.
Hypoxic-ischemic encephalopathy or myelopathy	An inciting event is frequently identified on history.
Infection/sepsis	Look for fever, other systemic signs of infection, laboratory abnormalities.

providing mechanical ventilation as needed, and administering continuous nasojejunal tube feedings. Intravenous and Foley catheters should be minimized to reduce the risk of any comorbid infections.[4]

Importantly, equine antitoxin, the preferred treatment for adult botulism infections, is not approved for infants because of the risk of anaphylaxis, lifelong hypersensitivity to equine antigens, its short half-life (5 to 7 days), and the lack of evidence as to a clinical benefit, even if babyBIG is not available.[5,7] Broad-spectrum anticlostridial antibiotics are also not recommended because they may result in a sudden increase in toxin release and rapid clinical deterioration.[2,7] In addition, aminoglycoside antibiotics for any other intercurrent illness should be avoided in cases of infant botulism because they cause presynaptic neuromuscular blockage, which may worsen botulism symptoms.[2]

With appropriate intensive care treatment, current case fatality of infant botulism is < 1% and full recovery is expected. Neurologic sequelae are rare, but systemic complications may arise related to prolonged intubation and aspiration.[3,6] Recurrence occurs in less than 5% of infants.[7]

References

1. Koepke R, Sobel J, Arnon SS. Global occurrence of infant botulism, 1976-2006. *Pediatrics.* 2008;122(1):e73-e82.
2. Tseng-Ong L, Mitchell WG. Infant botulism: 20 years' experience at a single institution. *J Child Neurol.* 2007;22(12):1333-1337.
3. Fox CK, Keet CA, Strober JB. Recent advances in infant botulism. *Pediatr Neurol.* 2005;32(3):149-154.
4. Long SS. Infant botulism and treatment with BIG-IV (BabyBIG). *Pediatr Infect Dis J.* 2007;26(3):261-262.
5. Arnon SS, Schechter R, Maslanka SE, Jewell NP, Hatheway CL. Human botulism immune globulin for the treatment of infant botulism. *N Engl J Med.* 2006;354(5):462-471.
6. Barnes M, Britton PN, Singh-Grewal D. Of war and sausages: a case-directed review of infant botulism. *J Paediatr Child Health.* 2013;49(3):e232-e234.
7. Domingo RM, Haller JS, Gruenthal M. Infant botulism: two recent cases and literature review. *J Child Neurol.* 2008;23(11):1336-1346.

SECTION V

CONCUSSION

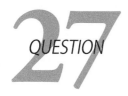

How Do I Know if a Child Has Had a Concussion?

Christina L. Master, MD, FAAP, CAQSM

Even with all the scientific advances in the understanding of the pathophysiology and epidemiology of concussion, the diagnosis of concussion still remains a clinical one. The essential elements for making the diagnosis of a concussion are (1) the history of a mechanism of injury, (2) subsequent symptoms that are typically seen in concussion, and (3) supporting physical examination deficits that are observed in concussion. The clinical history is probably the most helpful piece of information to you in making the diagnosis, and asking the right questions can point you in the right direction.

The first thing to establish is the mechanism of injury. One does not have to sustain a direct blow to the head in order to have a concussion; this is one of the most common lay misconceptions that make people think that a concussion has not occurred, when in fact, one has. Indirect forces transmitted to the head, such as a blow to the body that results in a whiplash effect on the head, are actually a common cause of concussion.[1] In addition, loss of consciousness is not necessary for a concussion to have occurred. Only approximately 10% of concussions are actually associated with loss of consciousness.[2] Oftentimes in the case of children, the injury event is unwitnessed and it takes some detective work on the parent's part to determine if there was an injury that may have caused the current presenting symptoms. Another consideration is the fact that sometimes incidental impacts, like bumping into a door, which may seem innocuous enough, in the right setting may actually be the cause of the current complaints that the child has. Remember, it does not always require a body-crushing football tackle or high-energy fall from the jungle gym to result in a concussion.

Licht DJ, Ryan NR, eds. *Curbside Consultation in Pediatric Neurology: 49 Clinical Questions* (pp 129-132).
© 2016 Taylor & Francis Group.

Table 27-1
Concussion Symptoms

Physical	Sleep	Thinking/ Remembering	Mood Disruption
Headache	Sleeping more or less than usual	Difficulty thinking or concentrating	More emotional
Nausea			Irritable
Vomiting	Drowsiness or fatigue	Difficulty remembering	Sad
Balance	Trouble falling asleep	Confusion	Nervous
Slowed reaction time			Depressed
Dizziness		Feeling mentally foggy	
Sensitivity to light		Feeling slowed down	
Sensitivity to sound			
Fuzzy or blurry vision			

Reprinted with permission from Master CL, Grady MF. Office-based management of pediatric and adolescent concussion. *Pediatric Annals.* 2012;41(9):1-6. Adapted from Pardini D, Stump J, Lovell M, Collins M, Moritz K, Fu F. The post-concussion symptom scale (PCSS): a factor analysis. *Br J Sports Med.* 2004;38:661-662.

Once a plausible mechanism of injury has been established, one can move on to detailing the clinical symptomatology that the child is presenting with. Again, depending on the age, there may be some challenges in elucidating the specific symptoms. Directed questions are often helpful as are close parental observations of their child; often the parents will note that the child is simply not acting like him- or herself. With older children and teenagers, they are often able to describe common symptoms in concussion such as headache, dizziness, and visual disturbances. With the heightened level of awareness of concussion today, many children and teens are able to recognize these symptoms as signs that they have a concussion. Some more subtle symptoms that a child may not think to report include sensitivity to light or sound, numbness or tingling, or feeling slow or foggy. Asking specifically about these symptoms is extremely important, otherwise you may miss specific symptoms that help direct you to the diagnosis of concussion. For younger children who may have more difficulty finding the words to describe how they are feeling, often parental report is essential. Besides the common symptoms of headache and dizziness, the younger children may have more issues that parents observe, such as emotional outbursts, either crying or fighting. Teenagers may notice symptoms that affect their main area of work—school. They often complain of memory or concentration problems or differences in how they are able to retain or recall information compared to before the injury. In general, the symptoms can be thought of as falling within the categories of physical, sleep-related, thinking-related, or emotional[3] (Table 27-1). Attention to all of these symptoms will be time well spent during your visit.

With all of the advances in understanding concussion, an increased awareness of the physical examination deficits found in concussion has also emerged. We all remember the days when a physician would say to a patient, "I think you have a concussion, but your physical exam is normal." In many cases, the physical exam is not normal; the physician was just not trained to look for specific deficits seen in concussion. If you haven't seen a concussion recently, it probably has seen you! In addition to the standard neurological exam that often can appear normal in concussion, it is important to assess other areas that may not be typically evaluated. Balance is an area that is often significantly disturbed in concussion. Single-leg stance, tandem stance, or tandem gait are often abnormal. Subtle changes can be brought out by having the patient perform tandem gait both forward and backward, with eyes open and closed, with the affected patient appearing very much like a drunk driver would appear on a field sobriety test.[4] In addition, subtle oculomotor deficits are present as well, but may not be observed unless you specifically attempt to elicit them. In particular, deficits in eye tracking are often noted in patients who complain of visual discomfort or other visual symptoms. Deficits of smooth pursuit can be elicited by having the patient track your finger rapidly moving from side to side. Horizontal and vertical saccades are tested by having the patient hold his or her head still while looking from side to side or up and down at 2 fixed objects. Children who have deficits with these activities will often complain of headache or dizziness with these maneuvers or will blink, pull away, or have their eyes well up with tears from the strain of performing these tests. Gaze stability deficits can be observed by having the patient focus on your thumb while nodding (vertical) and shaking (horizontal) his or her head, and these deficits are often associated with symptoms elicited with either running or reading, respectively.[5] Lastly, convergence insufficiency is often present, manifesting as the inability to transition visual attention from far to near; normal convergence is around 6 cm from the tip of the nose,[6] and in concussion it can be significantly increased to 10, 15, or even 25 cm or more. A simple method to assess in the office involves using a pen with some lettering, having the patient bring it toward the nose and stop when it is blurry or double, and measuring the distance from the tip of the nose. Once you know to probe these areas of balance and vestibulo-ocular and oculomotor function (Table 27-2) and find deficits, you can have confidence that your physical examination reaffirms your clinical suspicion of the diagnosis of concussion.

References

1. McCrory P, Meeuwisse W, Johnston K, et al. Consensus Statement on Concussion in Sport—the 3rd International Conference on Concussion in Sport held in Zurich, November 2008. *Clin J Sport Med.* 2009;19(3):185-200.
2. Langlois JA, Rutland-Brown W, Wald MM. The epidemiology and impact of traumatic brain injury: a brief overview. *J Head Trauma Rehabil.* 2006;21(5):375-378.
3. Pardini D, Stump J, Lovell M, Collins M, Moritz K, Fu F. The post-concussion symptom scale (PCSS): a factor analysis. *Br J Sports Med.* 2004;38:661-662.
4. Riemann BL, Guskiewicz KM. Effects of mild head injury on postural stability as measured through clinical balance testing. *J Athl Train.* 2000;35(1):19-25.
5. Master CL, Grady MF. Office-based management of pediatric and adolescent concussion. *Pediatr Ann.* 2012;41(9):1-6.
6. Lavrich JB. Convergence insufficiency and its current treatment. *Curr Opin Ophthalmol.* 2010;21(5):356-360.

Table 27-2

Specific Physical Examination Deficits in Concussion

Physical Examination Elements	How to Perform Exam	Findings
Dysmetria	Finger-nose-finger with examiner's finger moving horizontally	Slow reaction time, past pointing
Nystagmus	Examiner's finger moving horizontally progressively more rapidly, stopping centrally	Unable to visually track, beats of nystagmus at center of visual field
Smooth pursuits	Examiner's finger moving horizontally progressively more rapidly	Unable to visually track, jerky, jumpy movements, provokes symptoms such as headache, dizziness, eye fatigue, signs such as tearing
Saccades	Examiner's fingers held at shoulder-width or forehead to chin distance to test horizontally and vertically	Unable to perform or can perform only a few repetitions before symptoms or signs provoked as above
Gaze stability	Patient fixes gaze on examiner's thumb while nodding and then shaking head	Unable to perform or can perform only a few repetitions before symptoms or signs provoked as above
Convergence insufficiency	Patient takes a pen with letters and holds at arm's length and brings toward the nose until becomes blurry/double	Letters become blurry or double at >6 cm from the tip of nose
Balance	Tandem heel-toe gait forward and backward with eyes open and closed	Raises arms for stability or widens gait or has extreme truncal swaying without normal righting

Reprinted with permission from Master CL, Grady MF. Office-based management of pediatric and adolescent concussion. *Pediatric Annals*. 2012;41(9):1-6.

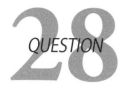

WHAT IS THE ROLE FOR HEAD IMAGING IN SUSPECTED CONCUSSION?

Matthew P. Kirschen, MD, PhD and Ronald F. Marchese, MD

The Centers for Disease Control and Prevention (CDC) estimates that 1.6 to 3.8 million sports-related concussions occur each year in the United States. More than half of sports-related concussions occur during football; however, impacts to the head are also common in other contact sports, such as soccer, lacrosse, rugby, ice hockey, and basketball. Sports-related concussions represent about 30% of all pediatric concussions that present to emergency departments (EDs); this percentage is higher (~40%) among adolescents aged 11 to 19 years.

Currently, there are no evidence-based guidelines to specifically address the role of head imaging after sports-related concussion. Consensus does exist within currently published guidelines that conventional structural imaging modalities, like computed tomography (CT) and magnetic resonance imaging (MRI), are generally of limited value in evaluating children and adolescents with suspected concussion. Imaging is not required for the diagnosis of concussion and contributes little to concussion evaluation and management.[1,2] Despite this, about 70% of children diagnosed with concussion in EDs undergo imaging, typically CT, during their evaluation.[3]

Athletes present to EDs after sports-related head injuries with a wide array of symptoms. Emergency physicians and consultants are faced with the challenge of determining which athletes require CT imaging to evaluate for central nervous system pathology (eg, intracranial hemorrhage) that may require surgical intervention, medical management, or inpatient observation. While neuroimaging is not recommended for routine sports-related concussions, urgent CT imaging should be considered to rule out structural brain injury in certain clinical scenarios.

Although no single study has produced guidelines with perfect sensitivity and specificity, several studies have shown that the presence of certain signs or symptoms is associated with an increased prevalence of intracranial injury. The CDC has published a list of neurological signs and symptoms to help guide the decision to perform head imaging (Table 28-1). These include, but are not limited to, a persistently altered mental status, a focal neurological deficit, evidence of skull

Licht DJ, Ryan NR, eds. *Curbside Consultation in Pediatric Neurology: 49 Clinical Questions* (pp 133-136).
© 2016 Taylor & Francis Group.

Table 28-1

Neurological Signs and Symptoms to Suggest Head Imaging Post-Concussion

- Headaches that are severe, worsen, persistent
- Seizures
- Focal neurological signs
- Visual changes
- Looks very drowsy or cannot be awakened
- Repeated vomiting
- Slurred speech
- Cannot recognize people or places
- Increasing confusion or irritability
- Weakness or numbness in arms or legs
- Neck pain
- Unusual behavior change
- Significant irritability
- Consider imaging if prolonged loss of consciousness (≥30 seconds)
  - Brief loss of consciousness (<30 seconds) should be taken seriously and the patient should be carefully monitored.

Adapted from US Department of Health and Human Services, Centers for Disease Control and Prevention. *Heads Up: Facts for Physicians About Mild Traumatic Brain Injury (MTBI)*. www.cdc.gov/con-cussion/headsup/pdf/Facts_for_Physicians_booklet-a.pdf

fracture on examination, or worsening symptoms or signs of clinical deterioration. Neuroimaging should be more strongly considered in children with underlying medical problems (ie, brain tumors, bleeding disorders, or epilepsy) who present with signs or symptoms of concussion, as these may also be indicative of a complication of their underlying condition.

It is helpful to identify those patients who are at very low risk for clinically significant structural intracranial injuries and do not need urgent CT imaging. A large, multicentered, prospective study to develop and validate criteria to identify such individuals concluded that pediatric patients with a Glasgow Coma Scale score of 15, normal mental status, and no history of loss of consciousness, vomiting, severe mechanism of injury, severe headache, or signs of a basilar skull fracture on physical examination do not need a head CT (negative predictive value = 99.95%).[4] Of note, these recommendations were designed by evaluating children with minor head injury of all types, not sports-related head injury specifically.

While CT is readily available and provides for early identification of post-traumatic intracranial pathology, it is associated with an increased risk of radiation-induced malignancies, which is of particular concern in children. If sedation is needed to obtain the study it adds additional risk for patients, particularly young children. In patients who do not meet high- or low-risk criteria, a period of observation in an ED has been shown to be safe and likely effective in reducing the number of head CT scans performed. The length of the observation period is controversial. One study has shown that the incidence of a delayed diagnosis of intracranial hemorrhage (≥6 hours after injury) in a patient without deterioration in level of consciousness was extremely low (0.57 cases per 100,000 patients per year).[5]

MRI offers significantly improved spatial resolution over CT and the multiple imaging sequences allow for detection of more subtle abnormalities like cerebral contusions. Specialized sequences like susceptibility weighted imaging (SWI) and diffusion tensor imaging (DTI) can be used in head-injured patients to detect lesions like microhemorrhages, white matter shearing, and diffuse axonal injury that can be missed by lower-resolution modalities. These findings do not require neurosurgical intervention, and it is unclear how they affect concussion management strategies as follow-up scans are typically not performed. DTI can identify microstructural white matter abnormalities within days after injury and has the potential to be a helpful diagnostic tool in certain situations; however, these findings currently have limited prognostic usefulness since no studies have correlated initial DTI results with long-term neurocognitive outcomes.

Determining whether a patient with a suspected or diagnosed concussion requires MRI scanning can be challenging, and no evidence-based guidelines or consensus recommendations exist to guide decision making. In the acute setting, MRI contributes little to concussion evaluation beyond CT. In the subacute and recovery phases of concussion, MRI may be useful if clinical symptoms suggest an alternative diagnosis such as a mass lesion. In our experience, MRI is of limited diagnostic valve for protracted concussion symptoms or post-concussion syndrome, but may be helpful in reassuring patients and their families as to the lack of intracranial pathology.

Although concussion results in microstructural changes in the brain, it is really more of a functional brain injury. Thus, functional neuroimaging modalities (eg, functional MRI [fMRI], positron emission tomography, MR spectroscopy, and single-photon emission computed tomography) may provide additional insight into mechanisms and pathophysiology of concussion-associated brain injury. For example, in a recent study using fMRI, football players who were never diagnosed with a concussion but sustained a significant number of subclinical impacts to the head demonstrated both neurocognitive and neurophysiologic impairments.[6] While these functional neuroimaging modalities at present are primarily used in the research domain, they may be employed in the future to individualize concussion assessment and management as well as monitor recovery. Patterns of functional injury may help predict recovery course and determine which patients are at greatest risk for more permanent injury with subsequent clinical or subclinical effects. Finally, these modalities may be helpful in assessing the effectiveness of therapies aimed at mitigating the effects of a concussion or accelerating recovery.

References

1. Halstead ME, Walter KD; Council on Sports Medicine and Fitness. American Academy of Pediatrics. Clinical report—sport-related concussion in children and adolescents. *Pediatrics.* 2010;126(3):597-615.
2. McCrory P, Meeuwisse WH, Aubry M, et al. Consensus statement on concussion in sport—the 4th International Conference on Concussion in Sport held in Zurich, November 2012. *Br J Sports Med.* 2013;47(5):250-258.
3. Meehan WP 3rd, Mannix R. Pediatric concussions in United States emergency departments in the years 2002 to 2006. *J Pediatr.* 2010;157(6):889-893.
4. Kuppermann N, Holmes JF, Dayan PS, et al. Identification of children at very low risk of clinically-important brain injuries after head trauma: a prospective cohort study. *Lancet.* 2009;374(9696):1160-1170.

5. Hamilton M, Mrazik M, Johnson DW. Incidence of delayed intracranial hemorrhage in children after uncompli-cated minor head injuries. *Pediatrics.* 2010;126(1):e33-e39.
6. Talavage TM, Nauman E, Breedlove EL, et al. Functionally-detected cognitive impairment in high school football players without clinically-diagnosed concussion. *J Neurotrauma.* 2014;31(4):327-338.

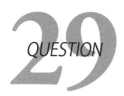

QUESTION

WHAT IS THE ACUTE MANAGEMENT AFTER A CONCUSSION? WHEN CAN A CHILD RETURN TO SCHOOL AND SPORTS?

Matthew Grady, MD, FAAP, CAQSM and
Christian Turner, MD, FAAP, CAQSM

Initial management following a possible traumatic brain injury is assessment of injury severity and determination of the correct diagnosis. Concussion is a clinical diagnosis that does not require imaging. In addition to concussion, other diagnoses could include cervical spine and intracranial injury. Red flags (Table 29-1) on the initial assessment require further evaluation—either additional imaging or prolonged observation.

The initial step in acute concussion management, following diagnosis, is prevention of additional injury. Whether it is interscholastic athletics or free play, children or young adults who sustain a concussion during play should not be returned to play or participate in any strenuous activities on the day of injury.[1]

A concussion is a traumatically induced injury of the brain. A shaking acceleration-deceleration force triggers a complex pathophysiological process, which results in a transient disturbance in brain function.[2] As this process progresses, animal models have demonstrated a neurometabolic cascade that results in alternations in ionic intracellular balance and metabolic brain function with accompanying microscopic axonal injury.[3] As such, concussion should not be viewed as a discrete injury, but as an injury process that evolves over a few days to weeks.

Very early in this process, there is an increased cerebral energy requirement, especially for glucose, to drive adenosine triphosphate (ATP)-dependent ion transport pumps and restore intracellular homeostasis. However, cerebral blood flow (and glucose delivery) is decreased immediately post-concussion and the recovery of normal cerebral flow is markedly delayed in children and adolescents compared to adults.[4] This creates an imbalance of energy requirements and energy substrate. This is frequently described as the "metabolic mismatch phase" of concussion. Clinicians should be aware that this metabolic mismatch phase may be more prolonged in younger patients compared to older adolescents.

Licht DJ, Ryan NR, eds. *Curbside Consultation in Pediatric Neurology: 49 Clinical Questions* (pp 137-140).
© 2016 Taylor & Francis Group.

Table 29-1

Red Flags in Concussion Evaluation

- Focal neurological deficit
- Vomiting ≥ 2
- Severe headache
- Significant alteration of mental status
- Suspected skull fracture
- Suspected cervical spine injury
- Loss of consciousness (> 1 minute more concerning)
- Prolonged amnesia (more than a few minutes)
- Dangerous mechanism of injury (car crash)

Starting from the moment a child is diagnosed with a concussion, the mainstay of initial management is "cognitive and physical rest." During the acute metabolic mismatch phase, the goal of management is to decrease overall cerebral energy requirements to minimize the mismatch. Forced exercise during this phase has been demonstrated to worsen the concussion.[5] Activities to avoid include running/jogging, biking, swimming, weight lifting, and sport participation including practice. Additional cognitive demands, such as schoolwork, video games, interactive computer programs, and text messaging may also exacerbate the injury and result in a delayed recovery. Early in the concussion injury, mental or physical exertion that makes symptoms worse should be avoided.

Return to School

During the early metabolic mismatch phase, there is some debate regarding how long to rest the brain from schoolwork. Since there is variability in injury severity, return-to-school decisions need to be made on a case-by-case basis. Individuals with severe symptoms or significant cognitive dysfunction may need to temporarily avoid all schoolwork. This may be true for the first few weeks in severe cases. With early rest, the majority (80% to 90%) of adolescent concussions recover within 4 weeks.

In our concussion practice, we advocate not going to school immediately following a concussion. This is not a universally accepted practice. Our rationale is that during the acute metabolic mismatch period, too much schoolwork and not enough rest may make the injury worse. We would prefer that students get adequate sleep immediately after the concussion. Sleeping 10 to 12 hours a day the first 1 to 2 days post-concussion is common. Maintaining a regular school schedule with early wake-up times may not allow sufficient rest.

As symptoms improve, schoolwork should be initiated slowly. This can be done while still symptomatic, but patients should be continuously monitored, and schoolwork scaled back if symptoms are worsening. As a practical matter, we have found it is much easier to initiate self-paced schoolwork at home in a quiet setting rather than at school. Transition back to the classroom is based on symptoms. In our experience, school readiness is generally based on the ability to complete at least an hour of schoolwork at home. School accommodations such as half days, extra

---

Table 29-2

Return-to-Play Process

1. Restart light aerobic activity once asymptomatic at rest and/or with school-work, heart rate < 70% maximum. No weight training
2. Sports-specific noncontact training activities such as skating, running
3. Noncontact sports-specific drills of increasing complexity, may start light weight training (resistance training)
4. Following medical clearance, allow full contact practice, participate in normal training activities
5. Full play, normal game play

Adapted from McCrory P, Meeuwisse W, Johnston K, et al. Consensus statement on Concussion in Sport—the 3rd International Conference on Concussion in Sport held in Zurich, November 2008. *Clin J Sport Med.* 2009;19(3):185-200.

---

time for assignments or tests, and frequent breaks may be necessary but are not usually required for more than a few weeks.

In individuals with prolonged symptoms (more than 1 month), there appears to be no additional advantage of rest. In a sense, the rules for return to school change. In our experience schoolwork should be initiated regardless of symptoms at this point. Options for schoolwork include homebound education or significant academic accommodations in school including decreased overall number of classes, adding study halls between classes as a rest period or decreased workload such as downgrading advanced placement/honors classes to regular classes.

If symptoms are limited to specific deficits, such as eye tracking or accommodation/convergence difficulties, then students need to limit reading and note taking. Preprinted teachers' notes, books on tape, large-print text, avoiding smart screens, and extra time for reading assignments are common school accommodations. Vestibular or vision therapy rehabilitation should be performed concurrently to address the underlying problems that are making return to full school difficult.

Return to Sports

The return to sports is a process that starts once a student has transitioned back to school. A return-to-play process (Table 29-2) is started after a student is able to fulfill a full day of school with no symptoms. In general, each step in the progression occurs over at least 24 hours. If an athlete is symptomatic with one step, he or she returns to the previous step.[6] Sports clearance should be seen as a process of completing all the steps rather than a set time after a concussion. To be cleared to return to play, an athlete should be asymptomatic (or at baseline) both with cognitive and physical activity and have a normal physical exam including balance and eye tracking.

In individuals with prolonged symptoms (more than 1 month), aerobic activity can be safely started even if an individual remains symptomatic.[7,8] At this point, initiation of aerobic activity is part of the rehab process, rather than part of the clearance process. Aerobic activity is performed to the threshold of making existing symptoms worse. As a practical guideline, an individual with a headache of 3/10 intensity could perform aerobic activity until the headache reaches a 5/10. Exercise at this point is continued until symptoms have returned to baseline. Clearance at this point should be guided by someone familiar with complicated concussion management.

References

1. Halstead ME, Walter KD; Council on Sports Medicine and Fitness. American Academy of Pediatrics. Clinical report—sport-related concussion in children and adolescents. *Pediatrics*. 2010;126(3):597-615.
2. Harmon KG, Drezner JA, Gammons M, et al. American Medical Society for Sports Medicine position statement: concussion in sport. *Br J Sports Med*. 2013;47(1):15-26.
3. Thompson HJ, Lifshitz J, Marklund N, et al. Lateral fluid percussion. Brain injury: a 15-year review and evaluation. *J Neurotrauma*. 2005;22(1):42-75.
4. Maugans TA, Farley C, Altaye M, Leach J, Cecil KM. Pediatric sports-related concussion produces cerebral blood flow alterations. *Pediatrics*. 2012;129(1):28-37.
5. Griesbach GS. Exercise after traumatic brain injury: is it a double-edged sword? *PM R*. 2011;3(6 Suppl 1):S64-S72.
6. McCrory P, Meeuwisse W, Johnston K, et al. Consensus statement on Concussion in Sport—the 3rd International Conference on Concussion in Sport held in Zurich, November 2008. *Clin J Sport Med*. 2009;19(3):185-200.
7. Gagnon I, Galli C, Friedman D, Grilli L, Iverson GL. Active rehabilitation for children who are slow to recover following sport-related concussion. *Brain Inj*. 2009;23(12):956-964.
8. Leddy JJ, Kozlowski K, Donnelly JP, Pendergast DR, Epstein LH, Willer B. A preliminary study of subsymptom threshold exercise training for refractory post-concussion syndrome. *Clin J Sport Med*. 2010;20(1):21-27.

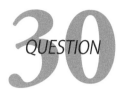

WHAT IS POST-CONCUSSIVE SYNDROME?

Matthew P. Kirschen, MD, PhD and
Maximillian H. Shmidheiser, PsyD, ABPP-CN

When evaluating or managing a patient who has sustained a concussion or mild traumatic brain injury, it is often challenging for practitioners to determine whether a patient's clinical symptoms are part of the concussion recovery process, or whether they have developed post-concussive syndrome (PCS).[1-3] Distinguishing between these 2 conditions can be difficult, especially since there is no universally accepted definition of PCS. The criteria for diagnosing PCS have been outlined by the *Diagnostic and Statistical Manual of Mental Disorders, Fourth Edition, Text Revision* (DSM-IV-TR) and *International Classification of Diseases, Tenth Edition* (ICD-10) (Table 30-1). Unfortunately, there is concern in the literature with regard to reliability and validity, as well as the lack of specificity and agreement between these diagnostic criteria.

The prevalence rates of PCS vary widely in the literature, which is likely because researchers use different definitions of PCS, in addition to using different patient populations and study methodologies. There is a continuum in concussion recovery that extends from the acute phase to more protracted symptoms, or PCS. In current clinical practice the point when the diagnosis switches from post-concussion symptoms to PCS is somewhat arbitrary and varies greatly among practitioners. It is relatively uncommon for concussion symptoms in adults to persist beyond 1 month (time criteria per ICD-10), and even fewer individuals have symptoms that persist beyond 3 months (time criteria per DSM-IV-TR). In our opinion, the management strategy during the recovery and rehabilitation from concussion is more important than determining the exact time PCS can be diagnosed. However, we diagnose PCS when concussion symptoms persist beyond a reasonable recovery period of several weeks. Recovery times can be longer for children and adolescents, and thus we reserve the diagnosis of PCS in children for when symptoms persist greater than several months.[4]

Licht DJ, Ryan NR, eds. *Curbside Consultation in Pediatric Neurology: 49 Clinical Questions* (pp 141-145).
© 2016 Taylor & Francis Group.

Table 30-1

Post-Concussive Syndrome Criteria

[a]International Classification of Diseases, Tenth Edition	[b]Diagnostic and Statistical Manual of Mental Disorders, Fourth Edition, Text Revision

• History of head trauma with loss of consciousness precedes symptom onset by maximum of 4 weeks
• Three or more symptom categories:
  1. Headache, dizziness, malaise, fatigue, noise intolerance
  2. Irritability, depression, anxiety, emotional lability
  3. Subjective concentration, memory, or intellectual difficulties without neuropsychological evidence of marked impairment
  4. Insomnia
  5. Reduced alcohol tolerance
  6. Preoccupation with above symptoms and fear of brain damage with hypochondriacal concern and adoption of sick role
	• A history of head trauma that has caused significant cerebral concussion (eg, with loss of consciousness, post-traumatic amnesia or seizures)
	• Neuropsychological evidence of difficulty in attention or memory
	• Three or more symptoms that last at least 3 months and have an onset shortly after head trauma or represent substantial worsening of previous symptoms:
	  1. Fatigue
	  2. Disordered sleep
	  3. Irritability or aggression with little or no provocation
	  4. Anxiety, depression, or affect lability
	  5. Headache
	  6. Dizziness
	  7. Changes in personality
	  8. Apathy or lack of spontaneity
	• The symptoms result in significant impairment in daily functioning that reflects a decline from previous level

[a]World Health Organization. *The ICD-10 Classification of Mental and Behavioural Disorders: Diagnostic Criteria for Research.* Geneva, Switzerland: Author; 1993.

[b]American Psychiatric Association. *Diagnostic and Statistical Manual of Mental Disorders, Fourth Edition, Text Revision.* Washington, DC: American Psychiatric Association; 2010.

PCS is labeled as post-concussional disorder (PCD) in the DSM-IV-TR. In the DSM-5 (2013), the neurocognitive and neuropsychiatric sequelae of traumatic brain injury, including concussion, are addressed within the framework of Neurocognitive Disorders (NCD).

Table 30-2
Clusters of Concussion Symptoms

Concussion Symptom Cluster	Symptom Examples
Physical	Headache, nausea, balance problems, dizziness, sensitivity to light, sensitivity to noise, or visual problems
Cognitive	Fatigue, drowsiness, feeling slowed down, feeling mentally "foggy," difficulty concentrating, or difficulty remembering
Neuropsychiatric	Irritability, sadness, or nervousness
Sleep	Difficulty sleeping or sleeping less than usual

Many hypotheses exist regarding what causes PCS symptoms to occur and persist, but a professional clinical consensus remains elusive. There is spirited debate regarding the degree to which these protracted symptoms are primarily physical or psychological. Some contend that PCS is due to central and systemic physiologic regulatory dysfunction, while others maintain that the development of PCS results primarily from psychological, psychosocial, and other issues that are nonspecific to concussion.[5] In either case, both neurophysiological and psychological factors are likely to be involved in the transformation of concussion to PCS.

The outpatient assessment and management of PCS is best undertaken through a multidisciplinary approach. The treatment team commonly includes a physician, neuropsychologist, and several therapists (eg, physical, vestibular, and vision) who all are trained and specialize in concussion management. Symptoms resulting from depression, post-traumatic stress disorder, chronic headaches, chronic pain, sleep dysfunction, or an interaction of several of these conditions may all produce symptoms similar to PCS. Thus, a systematic evaluation of each patient's concussion and its manifestations is crucial to obtain an accurate diagnosis and to initiate proper therapies.

The approach to assessing protracted post-concussion issues requires obtaining a detailed concussion history since clarifying etiological factors contributing to PCS is essential to informing appropriate treatment interventions. Questions should cover history related to prior concussions, headaches or migraines (including first-degree relatives), cognitive and physical development, sleep, and other neurological and psychiatric disorders. Next, comprehensive assessments of clinical symptoms, cognitive function, and balance are needed.

- Clinical symptoms: Numerous standardized symptom scales are available (eg, Post-Concussion Symptom Scale) and can be helpful if used serially throughout concussion recovery. Symptoms are often divided into 4 clusters (Table 30-2).[6] Since these measures rely on self-reporting and are not objective, they may be biased by underreporting (eg, for an athlete eager to return to play) or overreporting/exaggeration (eg, for a patient receiving secondary gain by playing the sick role or avoiding school). The patient's medical history, especially if there is a history of chronic headaches/migraines or pain or other neurological or psychiatric disorders should be considered when interpreting clinical symptoms.

- Cognitive functioning: Assessments can include traditional paper-and-pencil tests (eg, Trail Making Tests) or computer-based neuropsychological test batteries (eg, Immediate Post-Concussion Assessment and Cognitive Testing [ImPACT], Cogstate's Computerized Cognitive Assessment Test [CCAT], or Automated Neuropsychological Assessment Metrics [ANAM]), which have grown significantly in popularity and sophistication over the past decade. A more comprehensive neuropsychological evaluation can be helpful for refractory cases.

- Balance/ocular/vestibular dysfunction: Postural stability testing can provide a helpful approach to objectively assessing the motor and vestibular domains of neurologic functioning. Computerized dynamic posturography is the gold standard, but the Balance Error Scoring System (BESS) is a more practical balance assessment that can be administered in 3 to 5 minutes in the office setting. A complete eye motility exam including assessing eye tracking, gaze stabilization, accommodation, and convergence may uncover deficits that contribute to other symptoms like difficulty reading, balance problems, and headaches. Ocular and vestibular dysfunction may also occur in the absence of cognitive impairments.

The foundation of acute post-concussion management is physical and cognitive rest, and is discussed in greater detail in Question 29. Treating patients during their recovery from a concussion and with PCS requires a comprehensive management plan that incorporates rehabilitation in multiple domains, including cognitive, physical (eg, vestibular, headache, and vision), sleep, and psychological. These plans should include details encompassing home, school, social, and extracurricular activities including athletics. Management of PCS typically involves patient-, family-, and school-centered education that normalizes the symptoms and informs the patient of the likelihood of a good prognosis and full recovery with a proper rehabilitation strategy. Additionally, psychotherapy and possibly pharmacotherapy may be indicated to assist with symptom management. We maintain regular contact with patients undergoing rehabilitation for PCS, initially with frequent office visits and contact by a team member at least once every 2 weeks.

Managing PCS can be challenging, especially given the interconnectedness of symptoms and the complex biopsychosocial issues in patients' lives. Patients should be encouraged to resume their regular daily activity pattern as soon as possible after their concussion. It is recommended that students return to school following a period of cognitive rest and gradually increase the intensity and length of cognitive activities. The trajectory for increasing cognitive load should be individualized, and students should be encouraged to tolerate some triggering or exacerbation of their symptoms as the cognitive demand and time expectations are increased. School accommodations will almost always be required and can be facilitated through a Section 504 Plan or an Individualized Education Program. Medications (eg, amantadine) may help facilitate recovery of some concussion-related neurocognitive dysfunction and should be prescribed by physicians who have specialized training and experience with these neuropsychotropic agents.

After an initial period of physical rest, patients are encouraged to gradually resume exercise and fitness-related activities since research has shown that subsymptom threshold exercise may help to improve PCS symptoms.[7,8] Physical rest for a prolonged period or too little physical activity may contribute to PCS symptoms, such as a disrupted sleep-wake cycle, increased stress, irritability, boredom, and depression. Similarly, too much physical activity initiated too quickly after a brain injury can exacerbate symptoms and further prolong the recovery process. As with cognitive rehabilitation, we encourage athletes to tolerate a mild increase in their concussion symptoms during exercise before decreasing intensity. Physical therapists and athletic trainers can be helpful in designing exercise regimens that promote recovery. As long as any post-concussion signs or symptoms persist, we advise patients to abstain from high-risk activities, such as contact sports, cycling, and skiing. If a subsequent concussion occurs during PCS rehabilitation, it will likely result in new or more severe symptoms and a protracted recovery.

Post-concussion symptom scales, completed either at home or during clinic visits, can help identify symptom triggers and alleviating factors, recognize domains to guide therapy, and track recovery. Some clinicians recommend that patients complete post-concussion symptom scales on a daily basis. Other providers request that patients not keep a daily symptom diary because they feel that this process results in patients focusing more directly on symptoms rather than recovery. Headaches are the most common, and often the most protracted, PCS symptom and can be challenging to treat, especially for patients with a history of migraine or chronic daily headaches. Treatment strategies vary and include behavioral techniques for reduction of headache triggers (eg, adequate sleep, regular meals, activity pacing, and trigger avoidance), stress management, completion of a daily headache log (noting key information such as duration, location, and severity), and medications (see Question 22).

Patients with oculomotor impairments, such as eye-tracking difficulties or convergence insufficiency, should be assessed by an eye care professional who has training and experience in treating patients with concussion-related vision conditions. Likewise, patients with balance and vestibular dysfunction should receive an evaluation from a trained physical or vestibular therapist. Insomnia and sleeping difficulties are also common in PCS, and patients should be counseled regarding maintaining good sleep hygiene and may benefit from evaluation and intervention by a sleep specialist. Neuropsychiatric symptoms associated with PCS may respond to psychotherapy, stress management, and possibly medications to regulate mood or anxiety. A structured skills-based approach to psychotherapy such as cognitive behavioral therapy can be particularly helpful and has been shown to be beneficial in patients with PCS. Finally, while many of these therapies can be beneficial in facilitating recovery from concussion and PCS, caution is advised in recommending too many therapies as the time burden of multiple therapy sessions and medical appointments can detract from the ultimate goal of resuming regular school and extracurricular activities.

References

1. Jotwani V, Harmon KG. Postconcussion syndrome in athletes. *Curr Sports Med Rep.* 2010;9(1):21-26.
2. McCrea M, American Academy of Clinical Neuropsychology. *Mild Traumatic Brain Injury and Postconcussion Syndrome: The New Evidence Base for Diagnosis and Treatment.* Oxford, United Kingdom: Oxford University Press; 2008.
3. Prigatano GP, Gale SD. The current status of postconcussion syndrome. *Curr Opin Psychiatry.* 2011;24(3):243-250.
4. Barlow KM, Crawford S, Stevenson A, Sandhu SS, Belanger F, Dewey D. Epidemiology of postconcussion syndrome in pediatric mild traumatic brain injury. *Pediatrics.* 2010;126(2):e374-e381.
5. Silverberg ND, Iverson GL. Etiology of the post-concussion syndrome: physiogenesis and psychogenesis revisited. *NeuroRehabilitation.* 2011;29(4):317-329.
6. Kontos AP, Elbin RJ, Schatz P, et al. A revised factor structure for the post-concussion symptom scale: baseline and postconcussion factors. *Am J Sports Med.* 2012;40(10):2375-2384.
7. Silverberg ND, Iverson GL. Is rest after concussion "the best medicine"?: recommendations for activity resumption following concussion in athletes, civilians, and military service members. *J Head Trauma Rehabil.* 2013;28(4):250-259.
8. Leddy JJ, Kozlowski K, Donnelly JP, Pendergast DR, Epstein LH, Willer B. A preliminary study of subsymptom threshold exercise training for refractory post-concussion syndrome. *Clin J Sport Med.* 2010;20(1):21-27.

SECTION VI

WEAKNESS

31

HOW DO YOU EVALUATE
ACUTE WEAKNESS IN A CHILD?

Diana X. Bharucha-Goebel, MD

One major distinction in evaluating a child with acute weakness is differentiating between upper motor neuron vs lower motor neuron and peripheral causes. Upper motor neuron diseases affect the corticospinal tracts from their origin in the cortex to their termination in the spinal cord. These lesions typically present with asymmetric weakness often contralateral to the lesion, and result in weakness, hyperreflexia, and increased tone. Lower motor neuron disorders may involve the anterior horn cell, peripheral nerve, neuromuscular junction, or muscle fibers. Weakness due to lower motor neuron disorders tend to be more symmetric with decreased muscle tone and reduced deep tendon reflexes.

This chapter will provide a brief overview of potential causes of acute weakness in a child as well as the approach to the evaluation of acute weakness. The evaluation of the hypotonic infant and the evaluation of a child with progressive or chronic weakness is covered elsewhere (see Questions 24 and 25).

Differential Diagnosis

In Table 31-1, you will find a broad differential diagnosis both for "central" and "peripheral" causes of acute weakness that are grouped by localization along the neuroaxis.

Licht DJ, Ryan NR, eds. *Curbside Consultation in Pediatric Neurology: 49 Clinical Questions* (pp 149-155).
© 2016 Taylor & Francis Group.

Table 31-1
Causes of Acute Weakness

Upper Motor Neuron or Central Weakness	
Cortex	Stroke (thrombotic or hemorrhagic)
	Metabolic disorders
	Demyelination (acute disseminated encephalomyelitis, clinically isolated syndrome, multiple sclerosis)
	Intracranial tumor
	Todd's paralysis (transient focal weakness lasting minutes to hours following a seizure)
	Hemiplegic migraine
	Alternating hemiplegia of childhood
Spinal cord	Spinal cord trauma/compression
	Spinal cord ischemia or hemorrhage
	Infection (eg, epidural abscess)
	Transverse myelitis
Lower Motor Neuron or Peripheral Weakness	
Anterior horn cell	Poliomyelitis (rare in the United States but exists in other parts of the world)
	West Nile virus
Peripheral nerve	Guillain-Barré syndrome or acute inflammatory demyelinating polyneuropathy
	Brachial plexitis/brachial neuritis
	Acute intermittent porphyria
	Toxins (heavy metals, ciguatera fish poisoning, paralytic shellfish poisoning/saxitoxin)
Neuromuscular junction	Botulism
	Myasthenia gravis
	Tick paralysis
	Organophosphate poisoning
Muscle	Polymyositis
	Dermatomyositis
	Rhabdomyolysis (consider association with carnitine palmitoyltransferase II deficiency or McArdle's disease)
	Steroid-associated myopathy
	Critical illness myopathy
	Periodic paralysis (eg, hyper- or hypokalemic periodic paralysis)
	Medication related (isoniazid, zidovudine, magnesium sulfate)

Table 31-2

Differential Diagnosis of New-Onset Weakness by Timing of Onset

Acute Onset (Minutes to Hours)	Subacute Onset (Hours to Days)	Slowly Progressive
• Trauma • Seizure (with Todd's paralysis) • Stroke • Subarachnoid hemorrhage • Intracranial hemorrhage • Hemiplegic migraine	• Infantile botulism • Medications (heavy metals, organophosphate exposure) • Hemiplegic migraine • Epidural hematoma/abscess • Infection • Transverse myelitis • Acute disseminated encephalomyelitis/inflammation • Guillain-Barré syndrome • Tick paralysis	• Tumor • Dermatomyositis • Myasthenia gravis

History

Various questions in the history could help narrow down the differential and may suggest certain etiologies. Factors such as nature of the onset of symptoms, duration of symptoms, associated symptoms, and pattern of onset of weakness are all useful tools in the history of a child with new-onset acute weakness. The timing to onset of weakness may be useful in narrowing down the differential diagnosis (Table 31-2). In addition, medication and possible exposure history are critical.

Always elicit the timing of symptoms, specifically by asking the family when the child was last seen to be normal. Elicit whether symptoms were sudden in onset or gradual and progressive in onset. Generally speaking, sudden, new-onset weakness almost always warrants immediate medical attention, and most often will warrant immediate referral to the emergency room for evaluation.

Other important localizing signs in a patient with new-onset sudden weakness would be the presence of speech difficulties (either in understanding language, speech production, or both), neglect, accompanied sensory abnormalities, visual field cut, double vision, ataxia, difficulty swallowing, and shortness of breath. Other key points in the history of a patient with acute weakness include preceding trauma, presence of a headache, or preceding seizure. In a patient with focal weakness noted out of sleep, it is possible that the patient had an unwitnessed seizure during sleep, with subsequent transient Todd's paralysis. You would look for gradual return to baseline over minutes to hours, and a history of prior seizures or epilepsy. New-onset weakness and seizures in a patient without a prior seizure history also warrant immediate attention and neuroimaging. A history of weakness in a patient with associated migraine-like headache could suggest hemiplegic migraine; however, this is a diagnosis that should be made once more severe causes of headache and weakness such as intracranial hemorrhage or stroke are ruled out.

Accompanying symptoms are also useful. For example, loss of vision in one eye, especially with difficulty with color vision in that eye, could suggest optic neuritis and may raise your suspicion for a demyelinating cause for the child's acute weakness. The presence of dark, tea-colored urine suggests rhabdomyolysis, which can be seen in association with several metabolic causes of weakness including carnitine palmitoyltransferase II (CPT-II) deficiency and glycogen-storage disease type V (GSD5) or McArdle's disease. New-onset, acutely progressive poor swallowing, constipation, with weakening cry and descending weakness in an infant should prompt evaluation for infantile botulism (see Question 26).

Eliciting the pattern of weakness can also be useful. For example, ascending weakness along with back pain should suggest acute inflammatory demyelinating polyneuropathy or Guillain-Barré syndrome (see Question 32). Descending weakness in an infant, especially in the setting of constipation and poor feeding, may suggest infant botulism.

Examination

While it may seem tempting to focus one's attention immediately on the area of weakness, the practitioner must follow a systematic and complete approach to the neurologic examination of all patients with weakness. This should begin with a brief mental status examination to determine level of alertness, orientation, ability to follow simple commands, comprehension of speech, and intact expression of speech.

Pertinent aspects to the neurologic examination include the following.

CRANIAL NERVE EXAMINATION

- Ptosis and/or ophthalmoplegia (may suggest myasthenia gravis)
- Ophthalmoplegia
- Facial droop (central cortical causes of weakness—including stroke, demyelinating disease, hemorrhage)
- Afferent pupillary defect (optic neuritis, which may be associated with demyelinating causes of weakness)
- Papilledema

SENSATION

Sensation will typically be intact in patients with neuromuscular junction or muscle causes of weakness, but may be abnormal in nerve, spinal cord, or cortical causes of weakness. In neuropathic causes, consider dermatomal patterns of numbness in addition to the pattern of weakness. A sensory level (ie, spinal level below which there is a loss of sensation) suggests a spinal cord lesion or compression at that level. Loss of pin-prick and temperature with preserved vibration suggests anterior cord syndrome (anterior spinal artery stroke), whereas the inverse (loss of vibration, preserved pin-prick) suggests posterior cord syndrome (compression, inflammation, or vitamin B_{12} deficiency).

Table 31-3
Grading Muscle Strength

Grade 5	Muscle contracts against full resistance
Grade 4	Muscle strength is reduced, but muscle contraction can still move joint against resistance
Grade 3	Force generated to lift only against gravity, but not against resistance
Grade 2	Muscle can move only if the resistance of gravity is removed (can move within horizontal plane)
Grade 1	A trace or flicker of movement can be seen or felt in the muscle
Grade 0	No movement is felt or observed

GAIT

A broad-based or ataxic gait could suggest cerebellar abnormality; a sensory ataxia with proprioceptive loss (loss of joint position and vibration sense) suggests dorsal column spinal cord involvement perhaps in a patient with a spinal cord lesion or with transverse myelitis.

Motor Examination

MUSCLE BULK

This is likely to be normal in a patient with new-onset acute weakness, as opposed to those with long-standing weakness who may develop certain patterns of atrophy.

TONE

Evaluate the patient's passive resistance to movement (increased tone in a weak extremity can be seen in patients with upper motor neuron causes of weakness).

MANUAL MUSCLE STRENGTH

Assess the patient's ability to push against resistance using a 0 to 5 Medical Research Council (MRC) scale of motor strength (Table 31-3). The pattern of muscle weakness is very important in the evaluation of a weak child.

GENERALIZED WEAKNESS

This can be seen in patients with myasthenia gravis, periodic paralysis syndromes, and organophosphate disorders.

Paraplegia or Hemiplegia

This may indicate cortical or spinal cord lesions (hemorrhage, stroke, or demyelinating causes).

Proximal Weakness

This is typically seen in muscular or neuromuscular junction causes of weakness; diagnostic considerations include rhabdomyolysis, dermatomyositis, polymyositis, botulism, and myasthenia gravis.

Distal Weakness

Consider Guillain-Barré syndrome, chronic inflammatory demyelinating polyneuropathy (rare in the pediatric population), and West Nile virus.

Additional Testing

Careful history and examination should ideally be able to narrow down particular diagnostic considerations. Testing considerations include the following:

- Evaluate respiratory function with negative inspiratory force (NIF, normal is greater than −60) and forced vital capacity (FVC, normal range gauged by linear height) testing and trend these to determine if the patient is at risk of impending respiratory decompensation (this is of particular concern in patients with myasthenia gravis, Guillain-Barré syndrome, and potentially botulism if not treated early). NIF can be performed on infants who are crying, though timing of the measurement is critical and may take multiple attempts.

- Vital signs

- Urinalysis: In the event of rhabdomyolysis, patients could have myoglobinuria and attention to hydration status and renal function must be made.

- Skin examination: Evaluate for tick as cause of tick paralysis (due to neurotoxin from the Rocky Mountain wood tick or Eastern dog tick).

- Neuroimaging: Helpful in the evaluation of acute weakness thought to localize to cortical or spinal cord causes (suspected ischemia, hemorrhage, tumor, demyelination).

- Lumbar puncture: When considering the diagnosis of Guillain-Barré syndrome, a lumbar puncture can be helpful to look for an elevation of protein without pleocytosis (cytoalbuminologic dissociation).

- *Clostridium botulinum* toxin: Sent from stool (evaluation of infantile botulism), is often linked to nearby construction with soil-harboring spores.

- Creatine kinase level: May be useful in the acute setting when considering diagnoses such as dermatomyositis or polymyositis.

- Electromyogram (EMG): A nerve conduction study and EMG are not typically useful in the immediate diagnosis of most acute causes of weakness. Although not necessary to make the diagnosis and to initiate treatment for Guillain-Barré syndrome, an EMG may be useful in more atypical cases or for prognostic information.

- Acetylcholine receptor antibody: Evaluation for myasthenia gravis (elevated in up to 80% of patients with generalized myasthenia).

- Muscle biopsy: This may be useful in evaluating a patient with myositis, but otherwise will rarely be useful in the evaluation of new-onset acute weakness. The decision to biopsy will likely be made in consultation with a child neurologist or a neuromuscular disease specialist.

This chapter is meant to provide suggested etiologies and possible initial steps in the evaluation of a child with new-onset weakness. As mentioned previously, typically in many of these scenarios, a child will require evaluation in an emergency room or may require referral on an outpatient basis to a child neurologist for more specific workup.

Suggested Readings

Migita R. Etiology and evaluation of the child with muscle weakness. Up-to-Date. Available at http://www.uptodate.com/contents/etiology-and-evaluation-of-the-child-with-muscle-weakness. Accessed March 20, 2015.

Wolf H. Hypotonia and weakness. In: Zaoutis LB, Chiang VW, eds. *Comprehensive Pediatric Hospital Medicine.* Philadelphia, PA: Mosby; 2007:807-814.

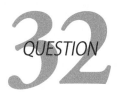

WHAT ARE THE CAUSES OF GUILLAIN-BARRÉ SYNDROME, HOW OFTEN DOES IT OCCUR, AND HOW DO YOU TREAT IT?

Jennifer L. McGuire, MD, MSCE

Guillain-Barré syndrome (GBS) is an acute inflammatory polyneuropathy classically characterized by rapidly progressive ascending symmetric weakness and areflexia. It is the most common cause of acute flaccid paralysis in infants and children year-round in the post-polio era,[1] with an annual incidence ranging from 0.34 to 1.3 pediatric cases per 100,000 children. While GBS may occur in all ages, it is less common in children under 2 years of age. In adults there is an increased risk of GBS in men compared to women (1.78 times)[2]; however, gender differences in children are not well defined.

GBS is a heterogeneous disorder with a number of different subtypes distinguished by specific clinical features (Table 32-1). While acute inflammatory demyelinating polyneuropathy (AIDP) is the most common variant in North America, demyelinating and/or axonal nerve pathologies may be seen, and all variants appear to be immunologically mediated. Autoimmune antibody production in GBS is probably primarily instigated by molecular mimicry.[1,2] Fifty to 82% of childhood GBS cases have an antecedent respiratory or gastrointestinal infection reported 3 days to 6 weeks prior to GBS presentation. The most common antecedent infection is gastroenteritis caused by *Campylobacter jejuni*, which occurs in 20% to 30% of demyelinating GBS cases in the United States and Europe[1] and many axonal and cranial nerve predominant cases worldwide.[2] Cytomegalovirus occurs in up to 10% of adult GBS cases in the United States, and is mostly associated with demyelinating forms of the disorder.[2] Varicella-zoster virus, *Haemophilus influenza* type B, herpes simplex virus, and *Mycoplasma pneumonia*[1,2] have also been reported antecedent to GBS. There was an increased rate of GBS following the 1976 influenza vaccine, but this has not recurred with any influenza vaccine since. Other epidemiologic risk factors include surgery and parturition.[3] GBS may also present in the context of hematologic malignancies such as lymphoma, as well as in the setting of seroconversion with human immunodeficiency virus (HIV).

Licht DJ, Ryan NR, eds. *Curbside Consultation in Pediatric Neurology: 49 Clinical Questions* (pp 157-161).
© 2016 Taylor & Francis Group.

Table 32-1
Common Guillain-Barré Syndrome Subtypes

Syndrome	Antibody	Important Features and Pathology
AIDP	None	Most common type of GBS (85% to 90%) in North America and Europe, with classic motor, sensory, and autonomic features of GBS. Demyelinating pathology.
AMAN	GM1, GD1a	Predominantly motor form of GBS, more common in Asia and South America. Axonal pathology.
AMSAN	GM1, GD1a	Similar to AMAN but with more sensory symptoms. Uncommon in children. Axonal pathology.
MFS	GQ1b, GT1a	Cranial nerve predominant form of GBS with descending weakness. Prominent clinical features include sensory ataxia, ophthalmoplegia, areflexia, and weakness.
BBE	GQ1b, GT1a	Brainstem encephalitis with encephalopathy, ataxia, ophthalmoplegia, and hyperreflexia. Probable clinical overlap with MFS.

AIDP: acute inflammatory demyelinating polyneuropathy; AMAN: acute motor axonal neuropathy; AMSAN: acute motor and sensory axonal neuropathy; MFS: Miller-Fisher syndrome; BBE: Bickerstaff's brainstem encephalitis.

Adapted from Rosen BA. Guillain-Barré syndrome. *Pediatr Rev.* 2012;33(4):164-170; quiz 170-171; Yuki N, Hartung HP. Guillain-Barré syndrome. *N Engl J Med.* 2012;366(24):2294-2304; and Ryan MM. Guillain-Barré syndrome in childhood. *J Paediatr Child Health.* 2005;41(5-6):237-241.

Clinically, most forms of GBS present as a rapidly progressive, bilateral, symmetric, length-dependent polyneuropathy causing weakness and sensory changes. While adults typically progress over 12 hours to 28 days before symptoms plateau,[2] 80% of children reach a clinical nadir within 14 days.[3] Many children also initially present with pain more prominent than weakness, although this pain can be diffuse and poorly localized causing children to appear irritable or encephalopathic.[3] Motor symptoms in children may present with refusal to walk or difficulty running or climbing.[1,4] In addition, unlike adults, 15% to 20% of children will initially have a proximal pattern of weakness, instead of the classic ascending pattern,[3] and sensory ataxia is common, mimicking common cerebellar disorders. Cranial nerve findings are seen in up to 50% of children,[1,3] with the bilateral facial nerves most commonly involved. As a result of these differences, up to two-thirds of preschool-age children with GBS may be initially misdiagnosed.[4] In general, a clearly defined sensory level, sudden-onset paralysis, persistently asymmetric weakness, ptosis, pupillary abnormalities, and prominent bulbar signs are uncommon in GBS and should prompt investigation of other etiologies.[1-3] A differential diagnosis of acute progressive bilateral symmetric weakness in children is presented in Table 32-2.

Over the course of their illness, 60% of children with GBS lose the ability to walk, and another 20% will need assistance. Seventy-six percent of children will have abnormal upper extremity function[1]; and 15% to 20% of children will require ventilatory support during their course of illness.[3,5]

Table 32-2
Differential Diagnosis of Acute Progressive Bilateral Symmetric Weakness in Children

Etiology	*Distinguishing Characteristics*
Tick paralysis	CSF is normal, symptoms resolve with tick removal. Ticks are commonly found at the hairline behind the ears.
Childhood botulism	Suspect with descending weakness, pupillary abnormalities, ophthalmoplegia, and early constipation. Diagnosis frequently made with NCS repetitive stimulation.
Myasthenia gravis	Commonly presents with fluctuating symptoms of proximal weakness and ptosis. Diagnosis frequently made with NCS repetitive stimulation.
Transverse myelitis	CSF typically demonstrates pleocytosis and elevated protein. Urinary or bowel sphincter dysfunction is common. EMG/NCS is normal. Early corticosteroids improve outcome.
Spinal cord compressive lesions	Urinary or bowel sphincter dysfunction, localized back pain, asymmetric weakness, and a discrete sensory level are common.
Toxic/metabolic neuropathies (lead, heavy metals, vincristine, organophosphates)	Exposure history or evidence of ingestion on expanded toxicology screen.
Infectious causes (enterovirus, West Nile virus, diphtheria)	Acute focal, asymmetric limb weakness, fever, pain. CSF typically demonstrates polymorphonuclear pleocytosis. Serologic testing may confirm the diagnosis.

CSF: cerebrospinal fluid; NCS: nerve conduction studies; EMG: electromyography.

Adapted from Rosen BA. Guillain-Barré syndrome. *Pediatr Rev.* 2012;33(4):164-170; quiz 170-171; Yuki N, Hartung HP. Guillain-Barré syndrome. *N Engl J Med.* 2012;366(24):2294-2304; and Ryan MM. Guillain-Barré syndrome in childhood. *J Paediatr Child Health.* 2005;41(5-6):237-241.

Bedside predictors of respiratory compromise include rapid progression of disease, abnormal pulmonary function, bulbar dysfunction, bilateral facial weakness, and dysautonomia.[5] Up to 25% of children will have serious autonomic dysfunction,[3] including widely fluctuant blood pressures and cardiac dysrhythmias. Marked bradycardia severe enough to cause asystole may occur, and pacing devices are therefore needed in rare cases.[3] Adult case series also reported fatigue in 60%, and vivid dreams, hallucinations, and psychosis in 33%[2] of GBS patients; the prevalence of these symptoms in children is unknown.

The diagnosis of GBS is based on clinical, laboratory, and electrophysiologic testing with a focus on exclusion of other possible symptom etiologies.[3] Lumbar puncture should be performed to rule out an infectious or neoplastic process. GBS classically demonstrates an albuminocytologic dissociation with elevated protein over 45 mg/dL in the absence of pleocytosis (< 10 cells/mm^3).[5] However, protein may remain normal for up to a week following presentation.[1,3] Magnetic resonance imaging (MRI) of the spine with and without gadolinium should be performed to rule out spinal cord compression, transverse myelitis, or other clear spinal cord etiology for weakness. GBS cases may demonstrate some gadolinium enhancement of the lumbar spinal nerve roots and cauda equina,[1,3] but this is not a specific finding.[6] Electrophysiologic studies (nerve conduction studies [NCS] and electromyography [EMG]) can help diagnose GBS and differentiate between primary axonal vs demyelinating subtypes. This exam should be performed after 1 week of symptoms for maximal sensitivity because 10% of children will have normal studies during the first week of illness.[1,3,5] Absent F wave (potentially the only early finding on NCS), prolonged distal latencies, conduction velocity slowing, and conduction block suggest demyelination, while reduced amplitudes of compound motor action potentials (CMAPs) without conduction slowing or prolongation of distal latencies suggest axonal injury. The ultimate diagnosis of GBS though is based on clinical criteria,[3] and therapy should be initiated even if supportive testing is normal given the possibility of false-negative results.[1]

Management of GBS is primarily supportive. Intensive care with cardiorespiratory monitoring should be initiated for those patients with rapidly progressive symptoms, bulbar involvement, reduced pulmonary vital capacity, flaccid quadriparesis, or autonomic instability. Mechanical ventilation should be considered prior to respiratory failure in individuals with vital capacities < 15 mL/kg, a partial pressure of oxygen (pO_2) < 70 mm Hg, or with significant muscle fatigue.[3] Nasogastric tubes should be placed if individuals are at risk for aspiration, and deep vein thrombosis prophylaxis should be used if weakness is predominant. Blood pressure medications should be used sparingly for hypertension, because they may induce sudden hypotension in the setting of blood pressure lability. Pain management typically requires opioid analgesics.[3] Finally, early physical therapy and rehabilitation once the patient passes the clinical nadir and begins functional improvement is critical for a timely recovery. During this time psychosocial support should also be provided.

Immunomodulatory therapy has been successful in reducing duration of mechanical ventilation, intensive care unit stay, and total hospitalization. Both plasma exchange (PLEX) and intravenous immunoglobulin (IVIG) within the first 2 weeks of symptom onset have proven effective while steroids have not demonstrated a benefit.[1] PLEX is typically administered using 5 exchanges over 2 weeks in children over 10 kg[3] and is thought to nonspecifically remove antibody and complement, thus reducing nerve damage and speeding clinical recovery.[2] IVIG is administered 2 grams IVIG per kilogram body weight divided over 5 days, and is hypothesized to work by neutralizing autoantibodies and inhibiting autoantibody-mediated complement activation, resulting in less nerve damage and faster improvement.[2] There has been only one trial comparing PLEX vs IVIG in children,[5] which demonstrated that children receiving PLEX had a small (2-day) improvement in duration of ventilation over IVIG patients, but there were no long-term differences in pediatric intensive care unit stay duration or short-term neurological outcome. Some providers feel that despite this small possible advantage to PLEX, IVIG is still preferred in children related to the technical issues surrounding PLEX catheter placement and large fluid shifts with exchange.[3] Clinical response may take up to 2 weeks after either therapy is complete. Following adequate therapy, more than 90% of children with GBS make a full recovery,[3] as compared to about 75% of affected adults.[2] The pediatric mortality rate is 1% to 2% and typically related to respiratory failure.[3] The remaining children may have residual sensory problems, fatigability, and poor coordination, but functional disability is uncommon.[1] Relapses of GBS are uncommon; however, some cases initially diagnosed as AIDP may actually represent the onset of a chronic inflammatory demyelinating polyneuropathy (CIDP), which requires different and often long-term therapy.

References

1. Rosen BA. Guillain-Barré syndrome. *Pediatr Rev.* 2012;33(4):164-170; quiz 170-171.
2. Yuki N, Hartung HP. Guillain-Barré syndrome. *N Engl J Med.* 2012;366(24):2294-2304.
3. Ryan MM. Guillain-Barré syndrome in childhood. *J Paediatr Child Health.* 2005;41(5-6):237-241.
4. Roodbol J, de Wit MC, Walgaard C, de Hoog M, Catsman-Berrevoets CE, Jacobs BC. Recognizing Guillain-Barre syndrome in preschool children. *Neurology.* 2011;76(9):807-810.
5. El-Bayoumi MA, El-Refaey AM, Abdelkader AM, El-Assmy MMA, Alwakeel AA, El-Tahan HM. Comparison of intravenous immunoglobulin and plasma exchange in treatment of mechanically ventilated children with Guillain Barré syndrome: a randomized study. *Crit Care.* 2011;15(4):R164.
6. Rabie M, Nevo Y. Childhood acute and chronic immune-mediated polyradiculoneuropathies. *Eur J Paediatr Neurol.* 2009;13(3):209-218.

SECTION VII

FOCAL NEUROLOGICAL DISEASE

WHAT ARE THE SIGNS OF A STROKE IN A CHILD? ARE THERE OTHER CONDITIONS THAT CAN PRESENT LIKE A STROKE?

Renée A. Shellhaas, MD, MS and Louis T. Dang, MD, PhD

Strokes are vascular events that result in a blockage of oxygen and nutrient delivery to brain cells, resulting in cell death (ischemia). Strokes are typically classified into 1 of 3 categories: (1) arterial ischemic stroke (AIS) is brain ischemia secondary to arterial occlusion; (2) hemorrhagic stroke comprises intraparencyhmal, intraventricular, and subarachnoid hemorrhages; and (3) venous stroke typically occurs in the context of cerebral venous sinus thrombosis (CVST) or cortical vein thrombosis. Arterial occlusion that spontaneously resolves can result in a transient ischemic attack, without findings of ischemia on magnetic resonance imaging (MRI) and with transient symptoms (typically < 1 hour in duration).

Although cerebrovascular disease is the second leading cause of death in adults, stroke is relatively rare in childhood (approximately 2.1 to 13.1 per 100,000 children per year). Nonetheless, stroke is as common as brain tumors in children. Because many other neurologic and non-neurologic conditions can present similarly, it is important for the clinician to suspect and recognize acute stroke, obtain urgent imaging for a prompt diagnosis, and institute acute management as indicated.

Signs of Stroke

Stroke usually presents with a sudden onset (80% of cases),[1] but symptom onset can evolve over hours to days. In many cases, there is a delay to stroke diagnosis, for multiple reasons, including difficulty in identifying focal neurologic problems in children, delays in bringing the child to medical care, lack of recognition of stroke by clinicians, and obstacles to obtaining neuroimaging.

Licht DJ, Ryan NR, eds. *Curbside Consultation in Pediatric Neurology: 49 Clinical Questions* (pp 165-169).
© 2016 Taylor & Francis Group.

Table 33-1

Typical Symptoms/Signs of Stroke in Children

Motor	Sensory	Cognitive	Nonlocalizing
Hemiparesis Facial weakness Persistent gaze deviation Focal seizures (with or without secondary generalization) Ophthalmoplegia Ataxia	Numbness Visual field defect Diplopia Sensory ataxia (lack of proprioception)	Aphasia (expressive or receptive) Depressed level of consciousness Neglect syndromes	Headache Nausea Vomiting Slurred speech Fatigue

You should suspect stroke when a child presents with an acute onset of focal neurologic symptoms (Table 33-1). The most common presenting symptoms of AIS are hemiparesis, facial weakness, slurred speech, and language deficits (impaired comprehension or fluency of speech). Less common presenting symptoms include sensory changes, ataxia, seizures, and visual changes (visual field deficit, diplopia, eye movement abnormalities, or persistent gaze deviation). In young or nonverbal children, visual deficits and sensory changes may not be detected because the child may not be able to describe the symptoms. Headache often occurs before, during, or after a stroke. Altered mental status can occur with any type of stroke, especially with posterior circulation AIS, but is less common with AIS than hemorrhagic or venous strokes. In a minority of patients with AIS, there is no clearly focal neurologic abnormality, and symptoms such as fatigue, drowsiness, or headache may be the only symptom present.

Children with hemorrhagic or venous strokes present with symptoms of increased intracranial pressure (depressed consciousness, vomiting, and headache) more often than children with AIS. These signs are often the primary presenting symptoms and they can progress rapidly, so these children typically require intensive care and aggressive interventions. Severe headache and seizures are common presenting symptoms in hemorrhagic stroke and CVST.

CVST can present with focal neurologic symptoms that are not confined to an arterial vascular distribution, and may not lateralize. Comorbid hemorrhage and secondary venous infarction can occur and may clinically resemble AIS. Typically, anticoagulation to recanalize the cerebral venous sinuses is warranted (even if there are minor parenchymal hemorrhages), to prevent further venous infarction and hemorrhage.

Neonates who suffer a stroke present with different symptoms than older children. Approximately 70% of neonates affected by a stroke present with focal motor seizures. Other symptoms include encephalopathy, apnea, hypotonia, asymmetric tone, asymmetric movements, and nonspecific symptoms such as irritability and poor feeding.[2]

Table 33-2

Differential Diagnosis of New-Onset (Focal) Neurologic Signs and Symptoms in Children

Cerebrovascular	*Cerebral, Nonvascular*	*Systemic*
Arterial ischemic stroke	Seizure/post-ictal states	Musculoskeletal abnormalities
Cerebral venous sinus thrombosis	Acute demyelinating encephalomyelitis	Drug toxicity
Intracranial hemorrhage	Cerebellitis	Delirium
Posterior reversible leukoencephalopathy syndrome	Complex migraine	Metabolic abnormalities
Vascular anomalies	Idiopathic intracranial hypertension	Conversion disorder
	Intracranial tumor	
	Intracranial infection	

Note: This list is not intended to be exhaustive. Rather, it is designed to convey the variety of clinical entities that are associated with focal neurologic signs and symptoms. Note that many items on the differential diagnosis can predispose to stroke.

Differential Diagnosis for Stroke

The differential diagnosis for an acute-onset focal neurologic problem is vast, and many disorders mimicking stroke must be considered (Table 33-2).

Seizures are very common during childhood and can manifest as a focal motor deficit, without the more commonly seen tonic or clonic movements. After a seizure involving the motor cortex, patients often have a post-ictal focal paralysis (Todd's paralysis). This should resolve over a period of minutes to hours.

Children with strokes commonly present with seizures (about 20% of cases).[1] Stroke should be suspected as the cause of a seizure in patients who have specific risk factors (eg, congenital cardiac abnormalities), but lack baseline neurologic problems that predispose them to seizures, or when a presumed Todd's paralysis does not resolve promptly.

Migraine variants are another common pediatric neurologic condition that may have associated focal neurologic signs and symptoms (eg, hemiplegic migraine, see Question 21). However, migraine is a diagnosis of exclusion.

Approximately 1 out of 5 children evaluated for possible stroke at one tertiary care center was found to have a stroke mimic.[3] Some mimics are categorized as benign conditions that are not expected to result in permanent neurologic deficits and which lack clinically significant structural abnormalities on imaging. These benign stroke mimics include musculoskeletal causes, somatoform disorder, and delirium. Other more worrisome conditions can also mimic childhood stroke, including posterior reversible leukoencephalopathy syndrome (PRES), vascular anomalies (eg, arteriovenous malformations, moyamoya disease), inflammatory diseases (such as acute disseminated encephalomyelitis), intracranial infection, metabolic stroke, tumor, drug toxicity, and idiopathic intracranial hypertension. Although a detailed clinical history is critical, no historical element can reliably differentiate benign from worrisome stroke mimics. Therefore, neuroimaging is usually required in order to make a definitive diagnosis.

Neuroimaging for Children With Suspected Stroke

Since history and examination alone are often insufficient for diagnosis, we recommend emergent neuroimaging in order to establish the correct diagnosis and guide therapy. Typically, it is fastest to obtain an emergent head CT (computed tomography) to examine for intracranial hemorrhage in cases of acute onset new focal neurologic symptoms. In cases of acute AIS, head CT may miss early lesions, and brain MRI with diffusion-weighted imaging (DWI) is the best modality to examine for acute ischemia and differentiate AIS from stroke mimics.[4] However, availability of emergent MRI scanning is often limited, and many children require sedation for MRI, which takes time and masks the neurological deficits. MR imaging can be expedited and performed without sedation in a child for whom there is high suspicion for stroke by obtaining a limited scan with T2-weighted and DWI sequences. When obtaining a complete MRI to evaluate suspected stroke, it is reasonable to also perform a MR angiogram of the head and neck and/or MR venogram to examine for arterial abnormalities as well as venous thrombosis. MR angiogram can provide accurate images of the arteries, without the radiation from CT angiography or radiation and invasive risks associated with conventional cerebral angiography.

CT angiography is often rapidly available and can identify arterial blockage. This modality may be preferred over MRI if acute intervention is being considered for AIS (eg, intravenous or intra-arterial tissue plasminogen activator [tPA]). Clinical safety and efficacy have not been well defined for these acute stroke treatments in children. Current guidelines advise against the use of tPA for children, except in the context of a clinical trial protocol. CT venography is also readily available, and can identify venous thrombosis, which may need to be treated with prompt anticoagulation.

Risk Factors for Childhood Stroke

Recognizing stroke risk factors aids in the differential diagnosis of children with new-onset focal neurologic deficits. The risk factors for childhood AIS are very different from those commonly diagnosed in adults (eg, hypertension and hyperlipidemia). Cerebral arteriopathies, congenital cardiac disease, and sickle cell disease are the most common pediatric stroke risk factors. The presence of these conditions in a child presenting with new focal neurologic signs or altered mental status should heighten suspicion for stroke.

However, many children do not have known risk factors at the time of presentation. Conditions such as inflammatory arteriopathy and thrombophilia are often diagnosed only after extensive evaluation in a symptomatic child. It has also been well described that infections, such as sepsis and meningitis, can be related to cerebral ischemia. Hemorrhagic stroke is often secondary to cerebrovascular abnormalities. If these cannot be seen on MR angiogram, more invasive conventional angiography may reveal the underlying lesion.

Summary

Stroke and stroke mimics should be considered in all children who present with the acute onset of focal neurologic symptoms or signs, especially for those with known risk factors for AIS, CVST, or intracranial hemorrhage. The differential diagnosis for focal neurologic signs and symptoms is broad, however. Brain imaging with CT and/or MRI is often key in the diagnosis, and ultimately the management, of children with stroke and stroke mimics.

References

1. Yock-Corrales A, Mackay MT, Mosley I, Maixner W, Babl FE. Acute childhood arterial ischemic and hemorrhagic stroke in the emergency department. *Ann Emerg Med.* 2011;58(2):156-163.
2. Shellhaas R, Smith S. Arterial ischemic perinatal stroke. *Journal of Pediatric Neurology.* 2010;8(3):251-258.
3. Shellhaas RA, Smith SE, O'Tool E, Licht DJ, Ichord RN. Mimics of childhood stroke: characteristics of a prospective cohort. *Pediatrics.* 2006;118(2):704-709.
4. Jordan LC, Hillis AE. Challenges in the diagnosis and treatment of pediatric stroke. *Nat Rev Neurol.* 2011;7(4):199-208.

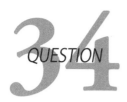

34

What Can I Tell a Parent to Expect About the Recovery From a Perinatal-Onset Arterial Ischemic Stroke? How About a Childhood-Onset Arterial Ischemic Stroke?

Lauren A. Beslow, MD, MSCE and Lori L. Billinghurst, MD, MSc, FRCPC

Questions around recovery and outcome after arterial ischemic stroke (AIS) are frequently encountered in neonatal and pediatric intensive care units and occasionally in the office setting after a diagnosis of stroke has been made. There are many clinical and radiological determinants of stroke outcome in children, including the underlying etiology, age at time of stroke, size and location of infarction, presence of hemorrhage, and comorbid conditions, such as congenital heart disease, coagulopathies, infection, head trauma, malignancy, and arteriopathy (Table 34-1).

Recovery after perinatal and childhood AIS can be variable, ranging from complete recovery to moderate to severe neurological deficits. As a general rule, clinical outcomes are better when compared to adults with similar strokes. Stroke outcomes have often focused on motor deficits and the ability to regain motor function that has been lost. However, other important aspects of recovery in children include language, sensory, cognitive, and behavioral functioning, as well as the ongoing and future risk of seizures or epilepsy (see Question 35) and recurrence risk of stroke. While we have many predictors of outcome, our ability to predict outcome is not well refined at this time. Each child's outcome is dependent on many factors and must be considered individually. Since some children recover fully or nearly fully, it is important to maintain a degree of optimism with parents when discussing prognoses. Parents may find support from several organizations in addition to that from their child's physicians and therapists (Table 34-2).

Licht DJ, Ryan NR, eds. *Curbside Consultation in Pediatric Neurology: 49 Clinical Questions* (pp 171-176). © 2016 Taylor & Francis Group.

Table 34-1

Risk Factors for Arterial Ischemic Stroke in Neonates and Children

Age Group	Risk Factors
Neonatal	• Chorioamnionitis • Inherited and maternally acquired prothrombotic disorders • Congenital cardiac disease • Meningitis • Sepsis • Cryptogenic

Childhood	• Arteriopathy
	   ○ Focal cerebral arteriopathy of childhood
	   ○ Post-varicella arteriopathy
	   ○ Moyamoya disease/syndrome
	   ○ Craniocervical dissection
	   ○ Vasculitis (primary or secondary)
	   ○ Post-radiation arteriopathy
	• Hematologic
	   ○ Inherited or acquired prothrombotic disorders
	   ○ Sickle cell disease
	   ○ Disseminated intravascular coagulation
	   ○ Thrombotic thrombocytopenic purpura
	   ○ Malignancy
	• Cardiac
	   ○ Congenital heart disease
	   ○ Valve abnormalities
	   ○ Intracardiac septal defect
	   ○ Intracardiac tumors
	   ○ Intracardiac thrombus
	   ○ Cardiomyopathy
	   ○ Arrhythmia
	• Infectious
	   ○ Meningitis
	   ○ Endocarditis
	   ○ Human immunodeficiency virus
	   ○ Syphilis
	• Rheumatologic
	   ○ Anticardiolipin antibody syndrome
	   ○ Systemic lupus erythematosus, other rheumatologic diseases with associated vasculitis
	   ○ Takayasu arteritis
	• Other
	   ○ Drug abuse, especially cocaine and amphetamines
	• Cryptogenic

<table>
<tr><td colspan="2" align="center"><u>Table 34-2</u>
Online Parent Support Resources</td></tr>
</table>

Organization	*Website*
Canadian Paediatric Stroke Support Association	www.cpssa.org
Children's Hemiplegia & Stroke Association	www.chasa.org
Hemi-Kids	www.hemikids.org
International Alliance for Pediatric Stroke	www.iapediatricstroke.org
Pediatric Stroke Network	www.pediatricstrokenetwork.com

Perinatal Stroke

Age of stroke onset seems to be a critical factor mediating the impact and recovery from stroke. Though previous models of brain development highlighted the role of plasticity as a buffer against deficits after brain injury, it has become increasingly clear that young brains are highly vulnerable to insult. Perinatal stroke includes fetal stroke (stroke before birth) and newborn or neonatal stroke (stroke at birth or in first 28 days of life.) Perinatal stroke may present in the newborn period (perinatal stroke) with seizures or in the first year of life (presumed perinatal stroke) with delayed developmental milestones, early handedness, or hemiplegia.

Newborns and very young infants with stroke may not initially show any symptoms or signs given the immaturity of the brain. However, sensorimotor, language, and cognitive deficits may slowly emerge as the brain develops and children face new learning challenges and developmental milestones. Indeed, motor outcomes such as cerebral palsy are often not fully realized and characterized until a child is well into the second year of life. Motor deficits affect 30% to 40% of children with perinatal stroke, and predicting long-term motor outcome in the acute setting is difficult. However, diffusion-weighted magnetic resonance imaging (DW-MRI) can be helpful in this regard. Poor motor outcome is correlated with volume of positive diffusion signal detected in the descending corticospinal tracts (internal capsule, cerebral peduncle, basis pontis, medullary pyramid; Figure 34-1). The absence of positive diffusion signal in these areas favors a mild to normal motor outcome in neonatal stroke. Additionally, nearly all neonates with stroke involving the basal ganglia have hemiparesis.

For complex neuropsychological skills, early age of stroke onset seems to predict poor outcome. Children with perinatal stroke have lower full-scale intelligence quotient (IQ) scores at school age than older infants and children with stroke and may demonstrate significantly lower full-scale IQ scores, impaired working memory, and reduced processing speed when compared to published norms. Boys tend to fare worse than girls in this regard. Further, children with presumed perinatal stroke have lower full-scale IQ scores than children with perinatal stroke. However, this relationship is not entirely linear and seems to be related to location of the infarction: subcortical networks are particularly vulnerable in neonates while cortical regions are most susceptible between 1 and 5 years of life. Children with perinatal stroke also appear to be at risk for later social and attention problems.

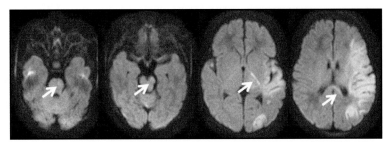

Figure 34-1. Axial magnetic resonance imaging from a 3-day-old with a perinatal stroke. Arrows demonstrate Wallerian changes (from left to right) in the white matter tracts of the descending corticospinal tracts in the pons, midbrain, posterior limb of the internal capsule, and in the splenium of the corpus callosum.

Childhood Stroke

There is also a high burden of neurological sequelae in childhood AIS. Up to 50% to 85% of survivors have permanent deficits including motor, language, cognitive, and social problems. Outcomes range from minor dysfunction that does not affect daily living to deficits that impair normal independent functioning. One study estimated that 40% of children with AIS have "good" recovery and 60% have "poor" recovery defined by whether the impairments affect daily function. Children are most commonly affected by hemiparesis and motor deficits (50% to 70%), and at least half have cognitive and behavioral difficulties. More than a third of children have language and speech deficits. It is important to recognize that mild deficits may not affect daily function or quality of life (QOL).

Outcome after childhood AIS can be predicted by Pediatric National Institutes of Health Stroke Scale (PedNIHSS) score. This score assesses clinical stroke severity in the acute setting and ranges from 0 (least severe) to 42 (most severe). The PedNIHSS score is predictive of neurological outcome gauged by the validated Pediatric Stroke Outcome Measure (PSOM) at 3 months and at 1 year after the stroke. Even when the PedNIHSS is not performed at presentation, the neurological examination documented by a neurologist can be used to create the score retrospectively. If that is not possible, it is reasonable to let parents know that clinically less-severe strokes are more likely to have better clinical recovery than more severe ones that have worse initial deficits. Decreased consciousness at presentation has also been associated with worse outcome. Radiological features that have been associated with poorer neurological prognosis include bilateral brain ischemia and arteriopathy. Larger infarction volume has been associated with worse neurological outcome in 2 studies, and one of these studies found a trend toward worse outcome with hemorrhagic transformation of the infarction.

Seizures and Epilepsy

In addition to neurological deficits, the presence of seizures and epilepsy and the need for ongoing treatment with antiseizure medications can affect the QOL and function of children after AIS. While more than 20% of children and 85% to 95% of newborns with AIS present with seizures at stroke onset, less is known about the need for anticonvulsant therapy in the recovery period and the development of remote seizures and epilepsy over time. However, some estimates of the prevalence of epilepsy after stroke are 15% to 25% (see Question 35).

Quality of Life After Stroke

School placement and QOL assessments are important for measuring the impact of the stroke on a child's life. In one study that investigated school placement, about 80% of children returned to a mainstream school, but nearly half of these children had a special educational need, and 40% required in-classroom help. Twenty percent of children attended a school for children with special needs. Several QOL studies have been performed in childhood AIS. In one study, QOL in childhood stroke survivors was lower than that of healthy children. Teenagers were particularly affected in the realm of peer interactions and emotional well-being. Parents or other proxy reporters rated the QOL both of school-age and teenage survivors of childhood stroke to be lower compared to the reports of parents and proxy reporters for healthy children. In another study, QOL related to school and play was most problematic for children with stroke, and QOL related to physical deficits and home environment was least problematic. Cognitive and behavioral deficits had a major impact on QOL. Another study both of children and neonates with stroke demonstrated that children with moderate-severe hemiparesis had worse health-related QOL when compared to those without hemiparesis or with mild hemiparesis. Furthermore, children with epilepsy had worse QOL than those without.

Stroke Recurrence Risk

Recurrence risk is very low in perinatal stroke and is estimated to be less than 1%. A few exceptions include children who have ongoing risk factors for stroke such as complex congenital heart disease (CHD) or blood clotting disorders. The recurrence risk for subsequent pregnancies for the same couple also appears to be extremely low. While this has not been well studied, one Canadian study of more than 400 children with perinatal stroke did not include a single case of recurrence within the same family. Further, one large multinational study of 347 infants with perinatal stroke failed to identify a single case of perinatal stroke in a sibling.

In contrast to the low recurrence risk of perinatal stroke, up to 19% of older infants and children with AIS will have a recurrent stroke by 5 years. For children with arteriopathy, this estimate may be as high as 66% by 5 years. Children who have recurrent stroke can accrue additional neurological deficits that affect their final neurological outcome and function. Therefore, a careful assessment of a child's recurrence risk is important. Certain stroke risk factors like moyamoya disease/syndrome, sickle cell anemia, and dissection have an especially high risk for recurrent stroke and for accrual of additional injury and deficits. Furthermore, children with underlying conditions such as CHD and malignancy may be exposed to prothrombotic medications and interventions that can affect stroke recurrence risk and thus final neurological outcome. While no randomized controlled trials exist for secondary prevention in childhood-onset stroke, in most cases antithrombotic agents are recommended by pediatric stroke experts. Antithrombotic agents commonly used include antiplatelet medications like acetylsalicylic acid and anticoagulants like low-molecular weight heparin and warfarin.

Recovery and Rehabilitation

Recovery following stroke is a dynamic process and rehabilitation likely leads to significant improvements in long-term outcomes. Given that the young brain continues to mature through adolescence, it is difficult to define the "recovery period" for children after stroke. To maximize a child's developmental potential and recovery, parents, physicians, physical and occupational therapists, speech and language pathologists, school personnel, and the child's community must take an active role. All children diagnosed with stroke should have a detailed assessment by health care professionals who specialize in rehabilitation. This interdisciplinary team will be able to determine the types of therapy a child could benefit from, the best locations where children can receive that care, and the duration of therapy.

It is important that rehabilitation therapy begin as soon as possible following a stroke. For children with residual deficits at the end of the acute hospitalization, careful assessments must be made in order to determine whether a child should be discharged to an inpatient rehabilitation facility or whether the child can receive outpatient therapy. Rehabilitation sessions work to improve functions that were affected by the stroke and assist in helping the child to adapt to physical or cognitive changes. Sessions may also include the development of skills that will be needed to be independent at school or at play. In addition, a formal neuropsychological evaluation and school assessments are often required to identify a child's strengths and weaknesses and to tailor a school program appropriate for the child's academic needs. Finally, serial neurological examinations and QOL assessments should be performed by a child neurologist or other experienced practitioner at regular intervals (often 6 to 12 weeks, 1 year, and yearly after stroke) to monitor the child's neurological recovery and ongoing needs.

Some children may not require any immediate therapy if a full or near-full recovery has been made in the hospital. Nevertheless, these children require close neurodevelopmental follow-up. Practitioners must be vigilant in identifying deficits that emerge as a child grows and develops and should expedite referral to appropriate therapists when issues arise.

Suggested Readings

Fullerton HJ, Wu YW, Sidney S, Johnston SC. Risk of recurrent childhood arterial ischemic stroke in a population-based cohort: the importance of cerebrovascular imaging. *Pediatrics.* 2007;119(3):495-501.

Ichord RN, Bastian R, Abraham L, et al. Interrater reliability of the Pediatric National Institutes of Health Stroke Scale (PedNIHSS) in a multicenter study. *Stroke.* 2011;42(3):613-617.

Neuner B, von Mackensen S, Krümpel A, et al. Health-related quality of life in children and adolescents with stroke, self-reports, and parent/proxies reports: cross-sectional investigation. *Ann Neurol.* 2011;70(1):70-78.

Roach ES, Golomb MR, Adams R, et al. Management of stroke in infants and children: a scientific statement from a Special Writing Group of the American Heart Association Stroke Council and the Council on Cardiovascular Disease in the Young. *Stroke.* 2008;39(9):2644-2691.

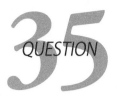

WHAT IS THE CHANCE OF DEVELOPING EPILEPSY AFTER STROKE?

Courtney J. Wusthoff, MD, MS

After a child receives initial care for stroke, attention quickly turns to understanding what consequences may follow. Families ask about the chance of ongoing motor or cognitive impairments. If the child had seizures as a presenting symptom, they may also ask about the risk of developing epilepsy. At the same time, the physician faces decisions about whether to continue any antiseizure medications used in the acute period, and whether specific follow-up is needed to screen for seizures or epilepsy.

First, the physician needs to clarify the difference between seizures and epilepsy. Few families would make this distinction up front. A seizure is a sudden episode of abnormal electrical activity in the brain; there are many reasons a person might have a seizure. When seizures are secondary to an identifiable cause, they are distinguished as symptomatic of the underlying problem. If a patient's only seizures are symptomatic of an acute problem, then the patient does not have epilepsy. For example, a patient may have multiple seizures on the day a stroke occurs, but this does not necessarily mean he or she will have epilepsy. Epilepsy is a chronic neurologic disorder characterized by recurring unprovoked seizures, or a tendency toward recurring seizures. While many children and neonates have symptomatic seizures around the time of a stroke, fewer go on to develop epilepsy.

Following stroke, about 6% to 9% of adults develop epilepsy. In those who do, the stroke has injured the brain in such a way that an ongoing tendency toward seizures remains. Strokes that injure cortex (as compared to strokes affecting only other parts of the brain) are more likely to result in epilepsy. In children, the overall risk of developing epilepsy after stroke is higher than in adults, ranging from 13% to 46%. Beyond this general estimate, there are factors that make a child more or less likely to develop epilepsy (Table 35-1).

In a retrospective series of 65 neonates and children with stroke, 54% (35 patients) had symptomatic seizures in the first week after stroke onset.[1] However, only 29% (19 patients) developed

Licht DJ, Ryan NR, eds. *Curbside Consultation in Pediatric Neurology: 49 Clinical Questions* (pp 177-180). © 2016 Taylor & Francis Group.

> ### Table 35-1
> # Risk Factors for Epilepsy After Stroke
>
> - Stroke involving cortex
> - Seizures during the acute hospitalization
> - Seizures starting > 7 days after stroke onset
> - Larger stroke size
> - Delayed presentation of presumed perinatal stroke

post-stroke epilepsy. Within this cohort, seizures starting more than 7 days after stroke onset were a significant risk factor. Of the 7 patients with seizures staring > 7 days after stroke, 6 (86%) developed post-stroke epilepsy. The authors also found that more patients with cortical strokes developed epilepsy (44%) than patients with subcortical (13%) or other strokes (0%). Similar post-stroke epilepsy rates were reported in a prospective study of 77 infants and children.[2] In this cohort, only 31% of patients had symptomatic seizures at presentation or during acute hospitalization. At 6-month follow-up, 24% overall had post-stroke epilepsy. All patients who developed post-stroke epilepsy also had seizures during the acute period; none of the patients without acute seizures developed later epilepsy. Additionally, a third, retrospective cohort of 62 infants and children with stroke describes similar results.[3] Many children initially had seizures around the time of stroke: 71% of infants and 21% of older children. Overall, only 15% had epilepsy at the time of follow-up. Finally, a prospective study of 46 neonates presenting with stroke in the newborn period found that 11% of babies had a single seizure during the follow-up period, and an additional 13% had epilepsy.[4] This study also found that newborns with smaller strokes were likely to remain seizure free, while those with large strokes were 6 times more likely to have post-stroke seizures or epilepsy.

When estimating the chance that a particular child will develop epilepsy after stroke, physicians should also take into account the clinical course to date. There may be a latent period of months or even years after stroke before a child presents with epilepsy. There is some suggestion that the ongoing risk of developing post-stroke epilepsy is lower after a child has remained seizure free for a few years; however, there is no cut-off time after which a child is guaranteed not to develop epilepsy. Similarly, context may be relevant to estimate epilepsy risk. For example, while the studies above found the overall risk of post-stroke epilepsy in children to be 13% to 29%, some specialist centers see rates of epilepsy after fetal or neonatal stroke as high as 46%.[5] This is largely because patients at highest risk are selectively referred to specialists; as a result, specialists see higher rates of problems after stroke. This is also true for patients with stroke diagnosed in retrospect. By definition, these are patients who seek medical attention because they had strokes severe enough to cause ongoing brain dysfunction, even though the stroke occurred months or years prior. One study among 45 children with delayed presentation and retrospective diagnosis of perinatal stroke found 38% developed epilepsy during follow-up.[6] None of these children had recognized seizures during the neonatal period around the time of presumed stroke, although neonates' seizures are notoriously subtle and might be missed if they self-resolve early. While physicians can provide an initial estimate of the chance of developing post-stroke epilepsy at the time of acute presentation, that estimate may need to be adjusted as time passes, based on the clinical course.

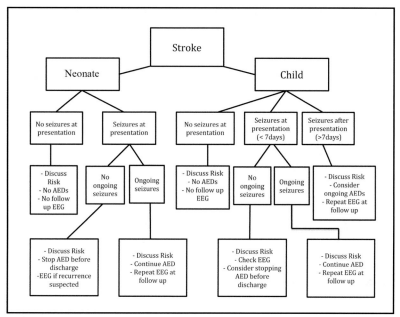

Figure 35-1. Suggested approach for evaluating epilepsy risk after pediatric stroke.

The literature provides evidence as a starting point for talking with families about the chance of developing epilepsy after stroke. When I talk to parents, I mention these numbers, and then explain whether I think a patient's risk is at the high or low end of the spectrum based on his or her particular combination of factors. If a patient did not have seizures around the time of the stroke, then the physician should also reassure parents that there is no reason to start an antiseizure medication after the fact, as most likely the child will not go on to develop epilepsy (Figure 35-1). Likewise, if there have not been any seizures, there is no reason to pursue follow-up electroencephalogram (EEG) studies. However, there is not enough evidence to define a single correct approach for children who have had seizures around the time of stroke, and are initially treated with antiseizure medicines. The potential benefits of preventing more seizures must be weighed against the potential risks of chronic medication. In neonates, I usually attempt to discontinue antiseizure medication prior to hospital discharge, but practices vary widely. In neonates and children, many neurologists find EEG useful to check whether epileptiform features have resolved as an indicator that antiseizure medicines can be weaned. There is no reason to check further EEGs after stopping medications in a child who remains seizure free. Discussing the specifics of a patient's case with a pediatric neurologist can be helpful in making decisions about medication in individual cases.

It is important to recognize that while many children have seizures around the time of their stroke, the majority will not go on to have epilepsy. A targeted review of the clinical course and neuroimaging can identify children at higher risk, and guide counseling for families along with a follow-up plan.

References

1. Morais NM, Ranzan J, Riesgo RS. Predictors of epilepsy in children with cerebrovascular disease. *J Child Neurol.* 2013;28(11):1387-1391.
2. Singh RK, Zecavati N, Singh J, et al. Seizures in acute childhood stroke. *J Pediatr.* 2012;160(2):291-296.
3. Lee EH, Yum MS, Ko TS. Risk factors and clinical outcomes of childhood ischemic stroke in a single Korean tertiary care center. *J Child Neurol.* 2012;27(4):485-491.
4. Wusthoff CJ, Kessler SK, Vossough A, et al. Risk of later seizure after perinatal arterial ischemic stroke: a prospective cohort study. *Pediatrics.* 2011;127(6):e1550-e1557.
5. Golomb MR, Garg BP, Carvalho KS, Johnson CS, Williams LS. Perinatal stroke and the risk of developing childhood epilepsy. *J Pediatr.* 2007;151(4):409-413.
6. Fitzgerald KC, Williams LS, Garg BP, Golomb MR. Epilepsy in children with delayed presentation of perinatal stroke. *J Child Neurol.* 2007;22(11):1274-1280.

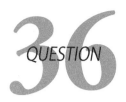

QUESTION

36

What Causes a Child to Have a Stroke?

John M. Binder, MD; Amanda L. Hollatz, MA; and
Timothy J. Bernard, MD, MSCS

Arterial ischemic strokes happen during 2 different timeframes during childhood: the neonatal period termed *perinatal stroke* and the childhood period termed *childhood stroke*. While the focus of this review is arterial ischemic stroke, strokes in children can also be hemorrhagic or venous. Perinatal ischemic stroke, occurring in a child less than 28 days old, has a prevalence of 1/4000 live births, and is much more common than childhood ischemic stroke. Children with perinatal ischemic stroke are diagnosed during 2 timeframes: some children present with seizures and/ or encephalopathy during the first few days of life, while others present at 4 to 8 months with weakness, hypertonia, and upper motor neuron signs on one side of the body. Magnetic resonance imaging (MRI) is essential to confirming the diagnosis of perinatal and childhood ischemic stroke, demonstrating evidence of ischemic damage in an arterial distribution that conforms to the clinical presentation. In neonates with a presentation of revealed hemiparesis at 4 to 8 months of life, we typically do not know exactly when the stroke occurred, leading to the classification of "presumed perinatal stroke" in these patients. Patients with childhood ischemic stroke, occurring at age 28 days to 18 years, usually present with an acute focal neurological deficit, such as hemiparesis, hemisensory loss, visual field cut, or aphasia. In children, there is typically no history of hypertension, diabetes, obesity, or other risk factors for atherosclerosis, as seen in adult ischemic stroke. Thus, the etiology of pediatric ischemic stroke is different from arterial ischemic stroke in adults. Ischemic stroke in neonates and children can be caused by many different diseases, but sometimes the etiology remains unknown.

In perinatal ischemic stroke, the source of embolus is often never found. Placental pathology can demonstrate evidence of an in situ clot suggesting paradoxical embolus from the placenta, so we always try to obtain placental pathology in these cases. In some children there will be a known congenital heart defect causing cardioembolic disease. In these children, a clot usually dislodges from the heart, travels to the brain, and lodges in an artery, causing ischemia. Although we usually

Licht DJ, Ryan NR, eds. *Curbside Consultation in
Pediatric Neurology: 49 Clinical Questions* (pp 181-185).
© 2016 Taylor & Francis Group.

recommend an echocardiogram in children with a perinatal stroke, the results are usually normal in children without a known history of cardiac disease. A patent foramen ovale is often found in perinatal stroke patients, but in general is not felt to be pathological and rarely changes management. In other cases, neonates are found to have a coagulation abnormality, such as protein C deficiency or antiphospholipid antibodies. Given the rarity of finding a severe clotting anomaly in these patients, the importance of coagulation workup in neonates is somewhat controversial. However, we typically recommend a hematology consult. Although recurrent stroke in this population is extraordinarily rare, the few patients who have recurrence will usually have a cardiac or thrombotic abnormality. Most babies with perinatal stroke, however, do not have an identified cause for stroke. While we know that a history of preeclampsia, infertility, prolonged rupture of membranes, and/or chorioamnionitis are all risk factors associated with perinatal stroke, exactly how these conditions are related to the etiology remains unknown. Similarly, there is often a history of delivery complications, including neonatal resuscitation, cesarean section, and 5-minute Apgar < 7. Given the low recurrence risk, unless an etiology is found for which therapy is indicated, we do not typically treat neonates with antithrombotic medicines. Supportive care and treatment of seizures, when present, is the standard of care.

Childhood ischemic stroke may occur from some of the same known causes as perinatal ischemic stroke, including heart disease or thrombophilia. Therefore, echocardiogram and thrombophilia evaluation are almost always warranted in children with ischemic stroke. Unlike perinatal ischemic stroke, abnormalities of the arteries of the brain and neck are a common cause of childhood ischemic stroke. A dissection of the extracranial arteries may cause clot formation and subsequent embolic stroke in children. Although some dissections occur spontaneously, many are associated with a rotational injury of the neck, such as dissection during rugby, chiropractor manipulation, climbing and reaching, landing on the head when playing on a trampoline, and falling off a skateboard. It is important to consider connective tissue abnormalities in these patients as well, especially if there is hyperextensibility on examination. Other cases of dissection can occur during more overt whiplash injuries, including those seen in a recent car accident. Increasingly, abnormalities in the intracranial arteries are also identified in childhood stroke. Recent studies have demonstrated that many children with stroke have irregular and narrowed intracranial arteries that may be contributing to the pathophysiology of their stroke. In rare instances, intracranial dissection may be the cause. In most cases, the intracranial arterial anomaly is considered a "focal cerebral arteriopathy," or unilateral stenosis and/or vessel irregularity of a large intracranial artery (internal carotid artery, middle cerebral artery, anterior cerebral artery) supplying the territory of infarct. While recent infection and inflammation is likely playing a role in causing these abnormal arteries to develop, we lack a complete understanding of the true etiology of these abnormalities. For this reason, the International Pediatric Stroke Study has an ongoing study exploring the role of infection and inflammation in children with stroke and focal cerebral arteriopathies, called the Vascular Effects of Infection in Pediatric Stroke Study. Initial workup of childhood stroke should include MRI of the brain, magnetic resonance angiography of the head and neck, echocardiogram with bubble, thrombophilia evaluation, and consideration of an inflammatory/infectious workup (Table 36-1). While the mainstay of treatment in childhood stroke is antithrombotic therapy, patients who are thought to have underlying inflammatory disease will sometimes also receive treatment with anti-inflammatory agents such as steroids. The choice of therapy and duration of treatment is not standardized and there is significant variability across the globe.

Table 36-1

Tiered Evaluation of Childhood Arterial Ischemic Stroke (Age 28 Days to 18 Years)

Primary Evaluation	*Secondary Evaluation Considerations*
Cerebral Imaging	
• MRI brain with diffusion-weighted, ADC, FLAIR, T1 and T2 images of the brain • MRA neck with T1 or T2 fat-saturation axial imaging • MRA head and neck with 3D time-of-flight (from the aortic arch through the circle of Willis); contrast-enhanced MRA should be highly considered in neck imaging	• CT angiography head and neck and/or conventional angiography head and neck
Cardiac	
• Echocardiogram with bubble • EKG	• Cardiology consult • 24-hour Holter monitoring
Thrombophilia Evaluation	
• Complete blood count • Factor VIII • D-Dimer • PT, PTT, INR • Antithrombin • Protein C activity • Free and total protein S antigen • FVL and/or functional activated protein C resistance assay • Prothrombin G20210A • Homocysteine level ± MTHFR • Lipoprotein (a) • Lupus anticoagulant • Anticardiolipin antibodies • Anti-β2GP-I antibody	• Hematology consult

(continued)

Table 36-1 (continued)

Tiered Evaluation of Childhood Arterial Ischemic Stroke (Age 28 Days to 18 Years)

Primary Evaluation	Secondary Evaluation Considerations
Inflammatory	
• ESR • CRP	• Rheumatology consult • Lumbar puncture (if safe) to include: whites, reds, protein glucose, VZV PCR, HZV PCR • ANA panel

MRI: magnetic resonance imaging; ADC: apparent diffusion coefficient; FLAIR: fluid attenuation inversion recovery; CT: computed tomography; MRA: magnetic resonance angiography; 3D: 3-dimensional; EKG: electrocardiogram; PT: prothrombin time, PTT: partial thromboplastin time; INR: international normalized ratio; FVL: factor V Leiden; MTHFR: methylenetetrahydrofolate reductase; Anti-β2GP-I: anti-β2-glycoprotein I; ESR: erythrocyte sedimentation rate; CRP: C-reactive protein; VZV PCR: varicella zoster virus by polymerase chain reaction; HZV PCR: herpes zoster virus; ANA: antinuclear antibodies.

Although most of these arterial abnormalities do not get worse over time, a small percentage of them progress. When arterial abnormalities in the distal internal carotid artery and proximal middle cerebral artery progress over time, then collaterals form and the disease is called moyamoya (Figure 36-1). The leading known cause of moyamoya disease is sickle cell disease, although many cases are idiopathic. Moyamoya has several tailored treatment strategies, with sickle cell-associated moyamoya patients receiving scheduled transfusions and idiopathic moyamoya patients undergoing revascularization procedures as the first line of therapy. Children with sickle cell disease, ages 2 to 16, should be screened annually with Transcranial Doppler (TCD) ultrasound in order to detect patients with early moyamoya and risk for stroke. TCD is a noninvasive and inexpensive screening tool used as primary prevention of stroke in children with sickle cell disease, identifying those children with high velocities in stenotic cerebral vessels.

As there are also multiple rare causes of childhood stroke including metabolic abnormalities such as Fabry's disease, chromosomal abnormalities such as trisomy 21, connective tissue disorders such as Ehlers-Danlos syndrome, or defined genetic syndromes such as PHACE syndrome (posterior cranial fossa malformations, facial hemangiomas, arterial anomalies, aortic coarctation and other cardiac defects, eye abnormalities, and sternal malformation or stenotic arterial diseases), consideration of evaluation by a childhood stroke specialist for tertiary evaluation should be made when an immediate cause is not found. Ultimately, however, the cause of perinatal and childhood ischemic stroke is often unknown, even following an exhaustive diagnostic workup.

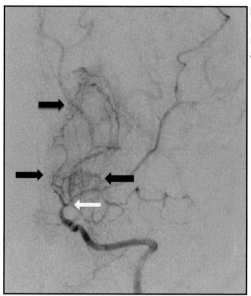

Figure 36-1. Conventional angiogram demonstrating moyamoya in a patient with internal carotid artery narrowing (white arrow) and classic puff-of-smoke appearance of collateral circulation (black arrows).

Suggested Readings

Bernard TJ, Manco-Johnson MJ, Goldenberg NA. The roles of anatomic factors, thrombophilia, and antithrombotic therapies in childhood-onset arterial ischemic stroke. *Thromb Res.* 2011;127(1):6-12.

Bernard TJ, Manco-Johnson MJ, Lo W, et al. Towards a consensus-based classification of childhood arterial ischemic stroke. *Stroke.* 2012;43(2):371-377.

Fullerton HJ, Elkind MS, Barkovich AJ, et al. The vascular effects of infection in Pediatric Stroke (VIPS) Study. *J Child Neurol.* 2011;26(9):1101-1110.

Goldenberg NA, Bernard TJ, Fullerton HJ, Gordon A, DeVeber G. Antithrombotic treatments, outcomes, and prognostic factors in acute childhood-onset arterial ischaemic stroke: a multicentre, observational, cohort study. *Lancet Neurol.* 2009;8(12):1120-1127.

Lee J, Croen LA, Backstrand KH, et al. Maternal and infant characteristics associated with perinatal arterial stroke in the infant. *JAMA.* 2005;293(6):723-729.

Nelson KB, Lynch JK. Stroke in newborn infants. *Lancet Neurol.* 2004;3(3):150-158.

SECTION VIII

VISION PROBLEMS

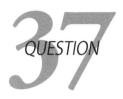

WHAT ARE THE IMPORTANT THINGS TO CONSIDER WHEN YOU SEE A CHILD WITH THE COMPLAINT OF VISION CHANGES?

Robert A. Avery, DO, MSCE

Children presenting to their primary physician with a complaint of vision changes can be daunting because of a variety of conditions it can represent. While a majority of cases require nonurgent consultation to a pediatric ophthalmologist, a few key historical and exam features can guide your referral timeline.

History

The approach to an ophthalmologic history is similar to any medical condition and should focus on features of location, duration, intensity, and exacerbating/relieving factors. Since most very young children cannot specifically describe their visual complaints, it is imperative to ask questions about the entire visual axis: eye appearance, type of vision complaint, and associated symptoms (like eye pain or headache). Starting with the eye itself, the overall appearance, presence of redness or inflammation, excessive tearing, and complaints of pain should be investigated. Has the child been rubbing the eye more often and what time of the day does it occur? Children who sleep with their eyes partially open will dry out their cornea and present with eye pain in the morning that is relieved later in the day as blinking adequately lubricates the eye. Frequent blinking can be the result of dry eye, seasonal allergies, or simple motor tics. Complaints of excessive glare suggest problems with the anterior portion of the eye.

When asked to describe their visual complaints, most children simply respond, "It's blurry." It is imperative to tease out whether their complaint is a mild and transient alteration in the clarity of the vision (ie, true "blurry vision"), a decline in the visual acuity, a decline in their visual field, or their description of double vision. Brief episodes of blurry vision that resolve within seconds after

Licht DJ, Ryan NR, eds. *Curbside Consultation in Pediatric Neurology: 49 Clinical Questions* (pp 189-193).
© 2016 Taylor & Francis Group.

Figure 37-1. Visual field deficit noticed in a coloring book from a child with an in utero stroke.

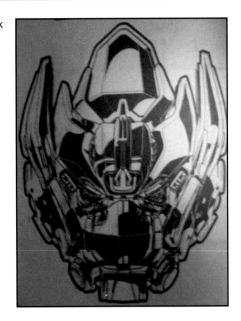

blinking or refocusing are typically benign. Historical features to inquire about when concerned about visual acuity loss include difficulty seeing the board at school, sitting close to the television/computer, or holding books close. Visually impaired children will also frequently adjust the position of their book/tablet to optimize their vision. Although fairly rare, progressive retinal diseases can manifest as difficulty seeing at night. The ability of children to ambulate well despite their complaint of vision loss should not distract the clinician from performing a thorough exam or referring to an ophthalmologist. Children with significant visual loss may also have impairment in depth perception. Parents will frequently describe a change in reaching skills, falling down stairs, or not being able to see 1 or 2 steps.

Visual complaints due to diplopia can present in a number of ways. To compensate for their ocular misalignment causing double vision, children may squint or close one eye, turn their head to one side, or even tilt their head. It is imperative to determine whether the child has monocular vs binocular diplopia. Binocular diplopia is caused by ocular misalignment that will resolve with covering either eye. If the complaint of diplopia persists while covering one eye, this is labeled as monocular diplopia. Monocular diplopia is typically an anterior segment (ie, cornea or lens) problem, but in children may be functional or simply their description of "blurry" vision.

Detecting visual field loss in children presenting with nonspecific visual complaints can be difficult. Unless a child is specifically describing absence of vision in the visual field, I tend to rely on historical features—especially in young children. Most children color or draw at a young age, so neglect of one part of the picture may suggest visual field loss (Figure 37-1).

Complaints of abnormal visual phenomena can be divided into 2 categories: positive and negative.[1] Bright colored spots, visual snow, or prism-like shimmering lines are considered positive phenomena and are frequently benign, although they can be associated with migraine headaches or seizures (rare). Positive phenomena should not obscure the child's vision, so asking whether he or she can still read or recognize faces is supportive of this symptom. Positive phenomena that are well-formed objects are considered hallucinations and should prompt a psychiatric referral. Absence of part or all of the visual field, described as "missing" or "black," are consistent with negative visual phenomena and can be a sign of significant pathology. Brief episodes (ie, 1 to 2 seconds) of negative visual phenomena, especially during an abrupt change in body position, are

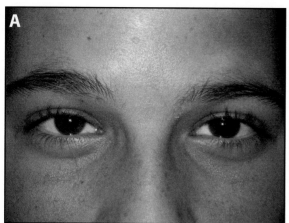

Figure 37-2. Pupillary light reflex in a near identical location on either pupil (A), but more lateral on the left pupil (B).

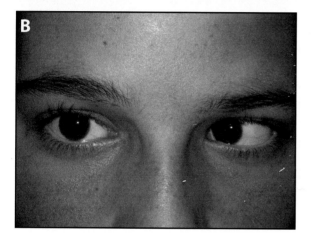

frequently benign. However, the persistence of negative phenomena should prompt urgent referral to an ophthalmologist or neurologist.

Examination

While the clinical history should help focus your examination, any complaint of vision changes requires the following components: external examination, visual acuity testing, visual field testing, pupil testing, ocular motility, ocular alignment, and fundus examination. The appearance of the cornea and conjunctiva can be made with a penlight or direct ophthalmoscope for redness, irritation, or abnormal appearance (ie, clouding of a cataract). Visual acuity is the most important test and must be completed by testing each eye separately. Using a standard office Snellen chart that includes figures and letters is ideal. Some young children may need encouragement to guess when they are unsure. Visual field testing can be conducted at arm's length, presenting fingers or toys in each of 4 quadrants, making sure to test each eye separately. Ocular alignment can be assessed by determining if the light reflex is positioned identically on both eyes (Figure 37-2). If diplopia or poor motility is suspected, these symptoms can be exacerbated by turning the child's head in the opposite direction while asking him or her to continue looking at the eye chart.

Figure 37-3. Unilateral optic nerve swelling in a child with elevated intracranial pressure.

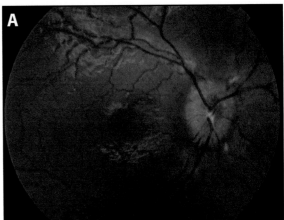

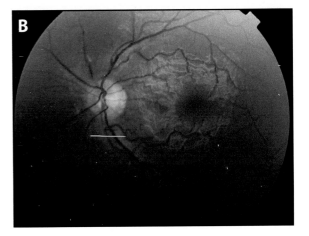

Performing a fundus examination on young, uncooperative children through an undilated pupil can be challenging. Viewing both optic nerves is required as optic nerve swelling can occur in only one eye (Figure 37-3). Mild and moderate papilledema can further complicate the examination, as the optic disc margins may be not observable.

Referral

The urgency with which to refer a child to a pediatric ophthalmologist or the emergency room depends on a number of factors. In general, any child with visual complaints in the setting of objective neurologic findings should be directed to the closest emergency room. Anterior segment complaints (eg, eye redness) may be cared for by the pediatrician or with the help of a phone consultation from a pediatric ophthalmologist. Children younger than 10 years of age with abnormal visual acuity believed to be related to refractive error (ie, a need for glasses) and who do not have other neurologic or ophthalmologic complaints can likely be seen within 4 weeks by a pediatric ophthalmologist. The acute onset of diplopia due to cranial nerve palsy requires urgent referral to a pediatric ophthalmologist or emergency room (Table 37-1). Most positive visual phenomena are benign, and in the setting of normal exam are nonurgent and

Table 37-1
Referral Algorithm for a Child With Visual Complaints

Complaint	Exam	Next Step
Blurry vision	Normal visual acuity and general exam	Observation, consider referral if it persists
Double vision	Strabismus	Urgent referral
	Cranial nerve palsy or associated neurologic signs/symptoms	Emergent referral
Vision loss	Visual field defect	Emergent referral
Small colored spots or visual snow	Normal visual acuity and general exam	Observation, consider referral if this persists

can be seen in 1 to 2 months if the symptoms persist. On the other hand, the acute onset and persistence of negative visual phenomena require urgent referral and may require neuroimaging, especially in the setting of concurrent neurologic symptoms including headache and ataxia.

Reference

1. Liu GT, Volpe NJ, Galetta SL. Visual hallucinations and illusions. In: *Neuro-Ophthalmology: Diagnosis and Management.* 2nd ed. Philadelphia, PA: Saunders Elsevier; 2010:393-412.

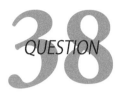

What Is the Evaluation of a Child With Optic Nerve Head Elevation (Papilledema)?

J. Michael Taylor, MD and Robert A. Avery, DO, MSCE

Exam Reveals Elevation of the Optic Nerve Head... Now What?

The acuity of this question ranges from emergent, as seen in papilledema from brain tumor, to a benign anatomical variant. The patient's clinical history and associated exam findings will help guide your decisions about subspecialty referral and need for prompt intracranial imaging.

What Is the Most Likely Cause of Optic Nerve Head Elevation? What Diagnosis Cannot Be Missed?

Optic nerve head elevation (ONHE) can be classified into 3 different groups (Table 38-1). In general the term *papilledema* is reserved for when elevated intracranial pressure causes ONHE (Figure 38-1). On the other hand, when the optic nerve is elevated from an inflammatory or infectious cause, we use the term *papillitis*. Certainly the finding of ONHE overlies the "don't miss" diagnoses such as tumors, meningitis, and impending threats of permanent vision loss (ie, idiopathic intracranial hypertension, also known as pseudotumor cerebri). While brain tumors are the most common cause of ONHE in children,[1] nearly all children have associated findings (eg, headache, ataxia) at presentation.[2]

Licht DJ, Ryan NR, eds. *Curbside Consultation in Pediatric Neurology: 49 Clinical Questions* (pp 195-199).
© 2016 Taylor & Francis Group.

Table 38-1
Differential Diagnosis of Optic Nerve Head Elevation in Children

Optic Nerve Finding	Causes
Papilledema	CNS tumor (most common)
	Idiopathic intracranial hypertension (second most common)
	Hydrocephalus: congenital, Chiari malformation, craniosynostosis
	CNS hemorrhage/sinus venous thrombosis
	Vascular anomaly: arteriovenous malformation, aneurysm
	Meningitis
	Medication: growth hormone, corticosteroids, minocycline, vitamin A derivatives
Papillitis/neuritis	Inflammatory: multiple sclerosis, neuromyelitis optica, systemic lupus erythematosus, sarcoidosis
	Vascular: ischemic optic neuropathy
	Infectious: *Borrelia burgdorferi* (Lyme), *Bartonella sp.* (cat scratch), *Toxoplasma gondii*, *Rickettsia sp.*, CMV
Pseudopapilledema/ anatomic	Optic nerve head drusen
	Myelinated nerve fibers
	Tilted discs

CNS: central nervous system; CMV: cytomegalovirus.

Figure 38-1. Papilledema with peripapillary retinal hemorrhages and developing macular star in a child with elevated intracranial pressure secondary to minocycline ingestion.

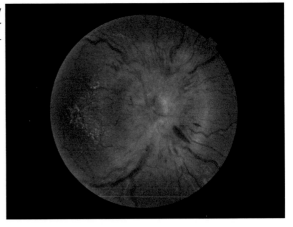

What Vision Symptoms Should I Ask About?

Inquiring about visual symptoms can be performed in a systemic manner—moving from the globe proximally to the retina, optic nerve, and ultimately the brain—and will be helpful in identifying an etiology. In addition to localizing value, this ordered approach to an ocular history prevents omission of important symptoms. Frequent and sustained eye redness may be suggestive of uveitis or iritis that accompanies autoimmune conditions affecting the anterior chamber as well as the optic nerve. Pain with eye movements can also indicate optic neuritis from an autoimmune or inflammatory condition. If the globe appears to be protruding out of the orbit (ie, proptosis, best seen by looking down at the globes from over the patient's head), then an orbital mass or inflammatory condition should be suspected. When proptosis is suspected, review of prior photographs can assess the chronicity of the finding (parents will frequently have pictures on their cell phones or social media pages). Changes in vision may be a symptom of ONHE. When interviewing the patient, focus on the clarity of the child's vision and whether he or she is displaying signs suggestive of visual acuity loss (eg, inability to read, sitting close to the television, trouble seeing the board at school) or visual field loss (eg, unexpectedly bumping into objects on the child's right side). Young children often have difficulty articulating vision changes and typically state things are "blurry." The loss of vision should be investigated in all children. Acute negative visual symptoms (ie, transient visual obscurations) are described as loss of part or the entire visual field and are frequently noted in elevated intracranial pressure. While transient visual obscurations quickly resolve, visual field loss from a tumor or stroke can be more chronic. Positive visual phenomena including flashing lights, colored lines/spots, formed visual hallucinations, or distortion of known images may be suggestive of migraine.

Beyond the clarity of vision, determining the presence or absence of diplopia (double vision) is imperative as this sign is highly suggestive of elevated intracranial pressure. Diplopia is caused by binocular misalignment resulting in the perception of 2 images, rather than one image. Images misaligned in the horizontal plane are frequently due to abducens (sixth) nerve palsy, whereas oblique or vertical diplopia is from oculomotor (third) or trochlear (fourth) nerve palsies. Families often notice a change in ocular alignment that can be confirmed by review of earlier photographs of the child. Squinting, covering or closing one eye when fixating, or a new head tilt suggests subtle misalignment. To differentiate "blurry" vision from true binocular diplopia, have the child occlude either eye with one hand. If the diplopia resolves, you have confirmed the symptom is secondary to eye misalignment. Monocular diplopia is rarely associated with pathology, having a strong association with functional disease.

What Neurological Symptoms Should I Ask About?

Consider obtaining this history in a head-to-toe fashion for localization and thoroughness. Sustained changes in behavior, sleep pattern, fatigue, ability to concentrate, and school performance can occur prior to onset of headache and emesis in patients with increased intracranial pressure. Symptoms suggestive of abnormal thyroid function, precocious puberty, accelerated/delayed growth, and excessive or secondary nocturnal enuresis often point to pituitary or hypothalamic dysfunction, such as occurs with midline tumors like craniopharyngioma. Ask if parents note a change in the child's smile or vocal quality. Less subtle are symptoms of excessive drooling, difficulty swallowing, and frank dysarthria. Extremity weakness or incoordination may be noted with changes in handwriting or hand preference. Ataxia may be seen in the trunk and extremities leading to clumsiness, falls, or other gait changes.

Are There Systemic Symptoms Associated With Optic Nerve Abnormalities?

Questions here should focus on suggestion of immune or inflammatory response. Screen for fever, rigors, weight loss, and other "B symptoms." Weight gain may also be seen with hypothalamic injury. The pattern of inflammatory changes in and around joints may suggest rheumatologic disease. Skin rash, erythema nodosum, and other integumentary changes are helpful clues to infectious and autoimmune disorders. Here is an opportunity to review recent travel and environmental exposures as well as family history. Medications known to cause increased intracranial pressure such as minocycline, growth hormone, oral contraceptives, corticosteroids, and vitamin A analogs should be reviewed.

What Am I Looking for on Exam?

A comprehensive physical exam should reveal pertinent signs associated with the differential above. Specific attention should be drawn to ocular and neurological deficits. Every exam should include testing visual acuity of each eye separately. Be aware that children with asymmetric vision loss may try to "peek" with their contralateral eye. Visual acuity is commonly spared in early ONHE; therefore, the absence of vision loss should not take you away from considering significant pathology. Visual field testing by confrontation in each eye separately is essential, but is notoriously insensitive to visual field loss.[3] Pupillary size and reactivity should be noted as well as asymmetries or differences in consensual responses. Observe extraocular movements and other brainstem signs for evidence of cranial neuropathy. Many pediatric brain tumors are in the posterior fossa, which reinforces the importance of identifying focal motor, sensory, and cerebellar signs that may localize here.

Are Blood Tests Helpful in Determining the Diagnosis?

Laboratory studies can assist in narrowing the differential diagnosis, and are most useful when a systemic disease is suspected. Geographic region and exposures (eg, new cat in the household) should be considered when diagnosing a suspected infection. Systemic inflammatory conditions including infection and autoimmune diseases may be screened for with erythrocyte sedimentation rate, C-reactive protein, complete blood count, and appropriate serologies.

Should I Arrange for a Lumbar Puncture?

Imaging is preferred prior to lumbar puncture to avoid conditions with a known risk of uncal or transtentorial herniation (eg, obstructive hydrocephalus). When safe to complete, every lumbar puncture should evaluate the opening pressure with the child positioned in the lateral recumbent position. Cerebrospinal studies should be directed toward the suspected etiology. If possible, collecting and saving an additional vial of 3 to 5 mL of cerebrospinal fluid may be helpful after the initial studies are performed. Although controversial, there is no proven benefit to draining additional cerebrospinal fluid from children with suspected intracranial hypertension.

What Imaging Study Should I Order?

Contrast-enhanced magnetic resonance imaging is the preferred study in most cases, but delays arise from scanner availability and arranging sedation in younger patients. As a general guideline, if the patient is acutely symptomatic with neurological or visual deficits, immediate referral to emergency care should be made. In this instance, computed tomography scan without contrast will typically identify lesions requiring emergent neurosurgical intervention. If no associated signs or symptoms are identified on thorough review, consider telephone consultation with your preferred child neurology or ophthalmology specialist prior to ordering additional imaging.

To Whom Should I Refer This Patient First?

Specialty care with neurology and ophthalmology should be arranged in order of provider availability if the child is asymptomatic. Alternatively, symptomatic patients should be urgently referred to the appropriate specialist or emergency department.

Summary

- Use clinical history and examination to narrow the differential diagnosis of ONHE.
- A battery of diagnostic tests, including intracranial imaging, is often required to establish a diagnosis.
- Subspecialty referral to pediatric ophthalmology and neurology providers can aid in ongoing management of optic nerve head edema.

References

1. Liu GT, Volpe NJ, Galetta SL. Optic disc swelling: papilledema and other causes. In: *Neuro-Ophthalmology: Diagnosis and Management.* 2nd ed. Philadelphia, PA: Saunders Elsevier; 2010:199-236.
2. The Childhood Brain Tumor Consortium. The epidemiology of headache among children with brain tumor. Headache in children with brain tumors. *J Neurooncol.* 1991;10(1):31-46.
3. Kerr NM, Chew SS, Eady EK, Gamble GD, Danesh-Meyer HV. Diagnostic accuracy of confrontation visual field tests. *Neurology.* 2010;74(15):1184-1190.

SECTION IX

VERTIGO

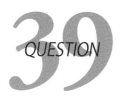

WHAT IS THE DIFFERENCE BETWEEN VERTIGO AND DIZZINESS? WHAT ARE COMMON CAUSES OF BOTH?

Alyssa Pensirikul, MD

"Dizziness" is a common complaint presenting to the pediatrician or emergency room physician. The symptom of dizziness is quite vague and can be used to describe several feelings of "fuzziness," balance difficulty, or lightheadedness, often mistaken for vertigo. Lightheadedness refers to presyncopal symptoms, or the feeling you get when you stand too quickly on a hot day. Vertigo is the sensation of spinning, either of oneself or of the surroundings. It is important to differentiate these 2 as they lead to 2 separate differential diagnoses. Vertigo (see Question 40) and syncope (see Question 2) are discussed in different chapters.

The anatomy of the sensation of balance is divided into peripheral and central components. Balance relies on input from the eyes and the peripheral sensory system that begins with pressure and touch receptors in the skin and stretch receptors in the joints. This sensory information is integrated in the cerebellum. The peripheral components of the vestibular system consist of the semicircular canals and the vestibule, which are located in the labyrinths of the inner ear. Angular acceleration of the head is picked up by the semicircular canals, of which there are 3 on each side of the head, to account for each plane of motion. The speed of the movement is proportional to the rate of firing of hair cells in the organ. The vestibule is made of the utricle and saccule and recognizes linear acceleration (such as sudden deceleration of a car).

As always, history is paramount in narrowing the differential and moving the patient toward the correct evaluation. Did the symptoms start acutely or insidiously? What was the patient doing when they started? Have they progressed or changed? What provokes the dizziness? Does the dizziness subside and after how long? Has there been any point since the symptoms started that the patient has been symptom free? Has the parent or caregiver noticed odd movements of the eyes (ie, nystagmus)? Has this type of dizziness ever occurred before (Table 39-1)?

What are accompanying symptoms: Is the patient nauseated or vomiting? Is there double vision and, if so, is it horizontal (objects aligned next to each other) or vertical diplopia (objects aligned

Licht DJ, Ryan NR, eds. *Curbside Consultation in Pediatric Neurology: 49 Clinical Questions* (pp 203-207).
© 2016 Taylor & Francis Group.

on top of each other)? (Any patient with diplopia should be referred immediately to the emergency room.) Is there headache and did it begin with the vertigo or is it secondary to the dizziness? Is there associated weakness or sensory changes? Tinnitus or hearing changes? Ataxia? Is there associated taste or odor or alteration of consciousness?

Further questions that might help elucidate an etiology would include: What makes the sensation worse (positional changes, blowing your nose, or bearing down during a bowel movement)? Was there a preceding illness? Was there preceding trauma, even if not overt (such as a rollercoaster ride, wrestling, or trampoline use)? Has the patient taken any medications or substances, including alcohol? Medications of interest would be benzodiazepines, antihistamines, aminoglycosides, seizure medication (particularly phenytoin or carbamazepine). Is there a family history of migraines, neurofibromatosis type 2, Ménière's disease, or von Hippel Lindau (cerebellar hemangioblastoma)?

The physical exam should include a full neurologic evaluation, particularly focusing on whether nystagmus is present and whether there are findings referable to the cerebellum such as dysmetria or ataxia. The Romberg test is asking the patient to stand with his or her eyes closed. The Romberg is a test of proprioception (the sensory integration of the dorsal columns, sensory information on joint position), vision, and the vestibular system. It requires 2 of the 3 to be intact. It does not test cerebellar function, and if the cerebellum is implicated in the process, then the Romberg test is not valid.

Causes of vertigo are divided into central and peripheral. Associated symptoms can help differentiate etiology (see Table 39-1). Generally, more severe symptoms such as significant nausea, vomiting, diaphoresis, and pallor are typically associated with peripheral vestibular dysfunction. Hearing loss (abrupt), tinnitus, or pain and pressure in the ear suggest a lesion of the labyrinth or eighth nerve (in the inner ear).

Peripheral Vestibular Dysfunction

BENIGN PAROXYSMAL POSITIONAL VERTIGO

Benign paroxysmal positional vertigo (BPPV) results when an otolith is displaced into one of the semicircular canals. This occurs following head trauma, infection, or as a result of aging. Because of the dislodged otolith, when the patient moves his or her head, the brain receives signals discordant with other incoming sensory symptoms and the patient feels vertiginous. The vertigo is typically of acute onset, short-lasting and recurrent, triggered by rolling over in bed or sudden head movement. There is associated nystagmus (jerky eye movements) and often nausea. It is diagnosed by description and confirmed by a positive Dix-Hallpike maneuver. Treatment is particle repositioning of the errant otolith with the Epley maneuver. Patient handout information on the Dix-Hallpike and Epley maneuvers can be found on uptodateonline.com.

LABYRINTHITIS

Labyrinthitis most often results from a viral infection or post-infectious inflammation. Rarely a bacterial infection from the middle ear or an extension of meningitis can cause labyrinthitis. Patients with classical labyrinthitis present with acute onset of vertigo that is constant, with nausea, vomiting, and unilateral hearing impairment. Chronic otitic infections can cause labyrinthine damage when a cholesteatoma develops. A cholesteatoma is a sac of keratin (produced by squamous cells) that gains access to the middle ear from the outer ear after repeated tympanic membrane perforations. Cholesteatomas erode surrounding tissues and can lead to a perilymphatic fistula. Symptoms of a fistula are provoked by maneuvers that increase pressure in the inner ear such as coughing, sneezing, or applying pressure on the external canal.

Table 39-1

Causes of Vertigo

	Tempo	Duration	Associated Symptoms					Related History			
			Nausea/ Vomiting	Hearing Impairment	Tinnitus/ Pressure	Altered Taste/ Smell	Altered Mental Status	Family History	Recent Infection	Trauma	Ingestion
Peripheral Vertigo											
Benign paroxysmal positional vertigo	Acute, Seconds	Intermittent/ provoked by position change	+++						±	±	
Vestibular neuronitis	Gradual, Days	Constant	+++						+		
Ménière's disease	Acute, Hours	Constant	+++		++			+			
Labyrinthitis	Acute, Days	Constant	+++	+					+		
Perilymphatic fistula	Acute, Days	Intermittent/ provoked by Valsalva	+++	+					+		
Central Vertigo											
Cerebellar stroke	Acute	Constant	±				±			±	
Acute cerebellitis	Gradual, Days	Constant							±		
Posterior fossa mass	Gradual	Constant					±				
Acoustic neuroma/ cerebellopontine angle mass	Gradual	Usually constant		+	+						
Toxin/ingestion	Gradual (hours), Hours	Constant	±				±				+
Migraine variant	Acute, Minutes to hours	Constant during spell	±					±			
Seizure	Acute, Minutes	Intermittent/ unprovoked				±	±				

MÉNIÈRE'S DISEASE

Ménière's disease is seen most commonly in patients with systemic inflammatory disorders like lupus, and is caused by an overaccumulation of endolymph that causes rupture of the labyrinth. It is uncommon in children. Symptoms include prominent tinnitus (ringing in the ear) and the sensation of fullness of the ear and hearing loss can precede the vertigo and tinnitus. Vertigo lasts 1 to 3 hours and tends to be repetitive for years and can lead to hearing loss. Treatment is symptomatic or with diuretics if more long-term management is required.

Central Causes of Vertigo

TRAUMA

Head trauma (such as that sustained during a sports concussion) can result in vertigo. Symptoms follow the trauma and tend to improve after weeks but can worsen with repeated concussion or with sudden movement of the head. Symptomatic treatment for severe symptoms with antihistamines or diazepam during the acute phase can be helpful. After the acute phase, some patients with persistent symptoms benefit from vestibular therapy.

MIGRAINES

Vertigo can be an aura to a migraine or part of the migraine itself. A migraine variant unique to children is known as benign paroxysmal vertigo. It occurs in young children ages 16 months to 2 years, and usually resolves by 4 years. Children complain of sudden dizziness ("the room is spinning") and nystagmus can be witnessed. The child refuses to walk and often to stand but, however, is not actually ataxic or dysmetric. Vomiting is uncommon. Episodes last hours to days and are often recurrent. It is helpful to obtain a family history of migraines. It is diagnosed after ruling out seizures with an electroencephalogram (EEG).

MASS LESIONS

Hearing loss and tinnitus with associated facial weakness would suggest a lesion in the ipsilateral internal auditory canal. Facial weakness and numbness, limb ataxia, hearing loss (slow and progressive), and tinnitus suggest an ipsilateral cerebellopontine angle mass. Involvement of cranial nerves (other than the seventh or eighth nerve, which together lie in the internal auditory canal) or long motor tracts localizes the lesion to the brainstem. Magnetic resonance imaging (MRI) is indicated in such concerns.

Epilepsy can present as episodic vertigo in which it can be the only symptom of a simple partial seizure or can precede a complex partial seizure. Sensations of taste or smell along with confusion or an altered mental status may also suggest a temporal lobe seizure. A routine or long-term EEG monitoring is indicated for patients with unexplained episodic vertigo without accompanying peripheral vestibular symptoms.

Though rare in childhood, a cerebellar or brainstem stroke should be suspected in a patient with an acute onset of vertigo with accompanying symptoms referable to the brainstem, cerebellum, or occipital lobes (in the distribution of the posterior circulation). Symptoms of diplopia, ataxia, vertigo, or vision loss should be followed with a thorough history of possible trauma that could result in injury or compression of the neck that could lead to dissection. The patient would require emergent evaluation. Vertebrobasilar insufficiency usually occurs in adults because of arteriosclerosis but may occur in a child with congenital arterial abnormalities like fibromuscular dysplasia.

CEREBELLAR ATAXIA AND CEREBELLITIS

Acute cerebellar ataxia and cerebellitis is a spectrum of illness that results from postinfectious autoimmune or parainfectious reasons. Further discussion can be found in Question 41.

If the history and physical do not lead to a secure diagnosis, it is prudent to strongly consider an MRI for further evaluation.

Suggested Readings

Cohen ME, Duffner PK. Vertigo. In: *Weiner and Levitt's Pediatric Neurology.* 4th ed. Philadelphia, PA: Lippincott Williams and Wilkins; 2003:277-281.

Fenichel GM. Lower brainstem and cranial nerve dysfunction. In: *Clinical Pediatric Neurology: A Signs and Symptoms Approach.* 6th ed. Philadelphia, PA: Saunders/Elsevier; 2009:364-368.

Rutka JA. Physiology of the vestibular system. In: Roland PS, Rutka JA, eds. *Ototoxicity.* Hamilton, Ontario, Canada: BC Decker; 2004:20-22.

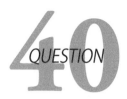

HOW SHOULD VERTIGO BE EVALUATED AND TREATED?

Alyssa R. Rosen, MD

Vertigo is understood as the subjective sensation of movement of the body relative to the environment. Patients may describe a feeling of the body spinning or rotating in space or of the environment spinning around the body. Vertigo can be accompanied by other related signs and symptoms (eg, imbalance, ataxia, nystagmus, nausea, or vomiting) or occur in isolation. Vertigo usually indicates a structural or functional disturbance of the vestibular system, which has both peripheral components (the labyrinth of the inner ear and eighth cranial nerve) and central components (brainstem, cerebellum, and cortex). The evaluation of vertigo must start with a thorough clinical history and careful physical examination, as this can narrow the differential diagnosis and direct further evaluation and treatment in most cases. The primary objective of the history and physical exam is to identify patients who require emergent evaluation for life-threating causes of vertigo and to distinguish central from peripheral vertigo. This will help determine the best initial diagnostic approach and most appropriate subspecialty referral (ie, neurology vs otolaryngology).

The first step in eliciting a vertigo history is to distinguish true vertigo from nonvertiginous dizziness (eg, lightheadedness, imbalance), which warrant separate evaluation. This may be challenging in the preverbal or nonverbal child but even very young children can often describe spinning ("like a merry-go-round") as distinct from other forms of dizziness. The next step is to determine the acuity of symptoms and identify any precipitating factors. Of particular interest are the relation of symptoms to postural changes, a recent history of trauma, prodromal or intercurrent illness, and any possibility of toxin ingestion or exposure. Next, an extensive query of associated symptoms should be reviewed, including the presence of fever or other infectious symptoms including neck pain and stiffness, cortical symptoms (eg, behavior changes, aphasia, focal weakness or altered mental status), cerebellar symptoms (eg, abnormal eye movements, discoordination, unsteady gait, imbalance), brainstem symptoms (eg, vomiting, double vision, slurred speech, difficulty swallowing, vocal changes), and peripheral vestibular symptoms (eg, ear pain

Licht DJ, Ryan NR, eds. *Curbside Consultation in Pediatric Neurology: 49 Clinical Questions* (pp 209-212).
© 2016 Taylor & Francis Group.

Table 40-1
Distinguishing Features of Central vs Peripheral Vertigo

	Central Pathology	*Peripheral Pathology*
Vertigo exacerbations	• Vertigo is constant	• **Vertigo is worse with head position change** • Improved with visual fixation (eyes open)
Mental status	• Normal or **impaired**	• Normal
Brainstem function	• **Abnormal eye alignment** • Voice clarity • **Tongue and palate strength and position** • Facial weakness (involving facial nerve nucleus)	• **Unilateral hearing loss** • Facial weakness (involving peripheral facial nerve)
Cerebellar function	• Dysmetria • Ataxia • Nystagmus (direction-changing or vertical)	• Ataxia • Nystagmus (pendular and **unidirectional**)

or fullness, tinnitus, hearing loss). The timing of symptoms and any palliating or provoking factors are also important. Specifically, changes in symptoms related to position, such as worsening with changes in body or head position, should be carefully queried, as this almost always points to peripheral pathology. Vertigo that is episodic or paroxysmal with periods of normal function in between attacks generally has a distinct differential diagnosis. That said, the first episode may be clinically indistinguishable from presentations of persistent vertigo and should be evaluated in a similar fashion.

Finally, a thorough physical examination must be performed. This should include orthostatic vital signs (especially if the patient does not draw a clear distinction between vertigo and lightheadedness), ear-nose-throat exam with special attention to any signs of infection or inflammation, and a complete neurologic exam. Key features of the neurologic exam and their relationship to central or peripheral dysfunction are outlined in Table 40-1. Certain maneuvers that test the vestibulo-ocular reflex can also be helpful. These could include having the patient fix his or her eyes on an object or the examiner's face while moving the head side to side or up and down, or asking the patient to hold visual fixation on the examiner's nose while the examiner twists the head quickly to one side and then the other (the head-thrust test). Loss of fixation of the eyes during the head-thrust test with a corrective saccade to the visual target to regain fixation is indicative of peripheral vestibular dysfunction. The Dix-Hallpike maneuver can be used to detect benign paroxysmal positional vertigo (BPPV). BPPV is rare in children, and the Dix-Hallpike maneuver requires practice and must be performed correctly to be diagnostically useful. It is therefore not practical for use in most general pediatric settings. Any maneuvers that involve manipulation of the neck should obviously be avoided in patients with recent trauma, neck pain, or any suspicion of vascular injury. Video demonstrations of both the head-thrust test and Dix-Hallpike maneuver are available through a quick online search.

Once the above evaluation is complete, a differential diagnosis can be generated and narrowed. As always, one should first consider the most dangerous and life-threatening conditions in the differential. Sudden-onset, persistent vertigo is much more concerning for a neurologic emergency than gradual-onset or episodic vertigo. Patients with symptoms that occur immediately following significant head or neck trauma, especially with severe headache, declining mental status, hemotympanum, vomiting, or those with brainstem or cerebellar signs on examination should be referred to the emergency room (ER) for emergent neuroimaging. Skull fracture, intracranial hemorrhage, and large strokes caused by injury to the vertebrobasilar circulation should be ruled out with an immediate noncontrast computed tomography (CT) of the head. If the head CT is negative but clinical suspicion remains, prompt magnetic resonance imaging (MRI) of the brain and vascular imaging of the head and neck (with MR angiogram or CT angiogram) is necessary to fully assess for stroke and vascular dissections. Advanced imaging of the inner ear may also be warranted (MRI with thin cuts of the temporal bone). Even without a history of trauma, patients with sudden-onset and persistent vertigo with brainstem or unilateral cerebellar signs on examination should undergo similar evaluation for stroke or hemorrhage as vascular dissections, embolic strokes, and ruptured vascular malformations can occur spontaneously in children. Posterior fossa and brainstem tumors, although they usually present with subacute and slowly progressive symptoms, may cause abrupt onset of symptoms due to hemorrhage or obstructive hydrocephalus. Other patients who warrant immediate ER evaluation are those with vertigo (or any other focal neurologic symptom) in the presence of fever, neck stiffness or altered mental status. These patients will need prompt head CT to rule out space-occupying lesions (eg, abscess) and increased intracranial pressure, followed by lumbar puncture and/or toxicological evaluation to rule out meningitis or ingestion. An MRI of the brain with and without contrast should be considered in such patients to assess for encephalitis, cerebellitis, and acute disseminated encephalomyelitis (ADEM).

If vertigo is subacute in onset or episodic and not accompanied by any of the above "red flags" on history or physical examination, a more measured diagnostic approach can be initiated. Here a clinical distinction between central and peripheral vertigo can be particularly useful. If vertigo is accompanied by ear pain or fullness, tinnitus, hearing loss, or abnormalities on otologic exam, the child should be treated for clinically obvious infections such as otitis media and otherwise referred to otolaryngology for further evaluation. An audiologic evaluation may be helpful as part of the assessment. Diagnostic considerations include mastoiditis, vestibular neuronitis or labyrinthitis, acoustic neuroma, BPPV, Ménière's disease, perilymphatic fistula, and Ramsay Hunt syndrome. Treatment will depend on the final diagnosis and should be directed by otolaryngology. If no obvious signs point to a peripheral cause of vertigo, the remaining central causes should be considered. The differential diagnosis can be narrowed by separating persistent from episodic vertigo. If vertigo is persistent (allowing for fluctuations with position changes, level of activity, stress, etc), the history should be probed for less-obvious precipitating factors. Vertigo is a common symptom after concussion and some concussions can be subtle and are not immediately identified (see separate section on concussion diagnosis and management in this text). A detailed medication history may reveal use of medications that can be associated with dizziness or even frank vertigo. If a clear historical precipitant is not identified or if significant abnormalities are present on neurologic exam, neuroimaging should be performed to rule out structural lesions such as tumors or the demyelinating lesions of multiple sclerosis. An MRI of the brain with and without intravenous contrast with thin cuts through the internal auditory canals will evaluate for the structural lesions that could lead to central or peripheral vertigo. Referral to a child neurologist may be considered at this point if imaging is negative or demonstrates brain pathology not better evaluated by another subspecialist (ie, neurosurgery or neuro-oncology). When vertigo is episodic, migraine and migraine equivalents are at the top of the differential diagnosis. Migraine accounts for 25% to 50% of vertigo syndromes in children.[1] Migrainous vertigo, or basilar migraine (see Question 21), can occur with or without the presence of headache, and migraine without headache is more common in children than adults.[2] In younger children, benign paroxysmal vertigo of childhood, a migraine equivalent, can present with attacks of vertigo accompanied by unsteadiness, nystagmus, nausea, vomiting, pallor, and diaphoresis lasting seconds to minutes. Consciousness remains intact and children can recall the episodes. They may fall asleep immediately following the attack.[3] Between attacks children are asymptomatic with a normal neurologic exam. A family history of migraine can frequently be elicited and many of these patients go on to develop typical migraines later in life.[1-3] Finally, vertigo in all forms can occur as part of a somatoform disorder. As with all somatoform disorders, a thorough investigation of physiologic causes should be exhausted prior to making the diagnosis. Treatment for each of the previous central causes of vertigo varies widely by diagnosis and discussions of these varied treatments are beyond the scope of this chapter. In general, children with vestibular symptoms from any cause (including somatoform disorders) may benefit from vestibular physical therapy and rehabilitation.

References

1. Casselbrant ML, Mandel EM. Balance disorders in children. *Neurol Clin.* 2005;23(3):807-829.
2. Jahn K. Vertigo and balance in children—diagnostic approach and insights from imaging. *Eur J Paediatr Neurol.* 2011;15(4):289-294.
3. Rothner AD, Menkes JH. Headaches and nonepileptic disorders. In: Menkes JH, Sarnat HB, Maria BL, eds. *Child Neurology.* Philadelphia, PA: Lippincott Williams and Wilkins; 2006:943-968.

SECTION X

ATAXIA

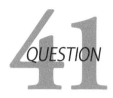

WHAT ARE COMMON CAUSES OF ACUTE ATAXIA IN CHILDREN?

David Bearden, MD

Overview

Ataxia may be secondary to cerebellar dysfunction, a disruption of sensory input to the brain, or vestibular dysfunction, and may be best approached by breaking it down by localization, associated symptoms, and time course.

Localization

Inputs to the cerebellum come from peripheral nerves and the vestibular system. Peripheral nerve inputs to the cerebellum (for position/vibration sensation) travel up the posterior columns of the spinal cord. Injury to either proprioceptive peripheral nerves or posterior columns causes a sensory ataxia, while injury to the vestibular apparatus in the inner ear or its inputs into the brainstem cause a vestibular ataxia. Clues to the localization of ataxia can be found in Table 41-1. The most common cause of ataxia in children is cerebellar ataxia, which will be the focus of this review.

Neuroanatomy of the Cerebellum

Ordering of movements takes place in the cerebellum, which integrates input from the sensory nerves and the vestibular apparatus to create smooth movements. The cerebellum can be divided into 3 parts: the midline vermis, which controls axial (midline) movements; the hemispheres, which control limb movements; and the flocculonodulus, which controls eye movements. Midline

Licht DJ, Ryan NR, eds. *Curbside Consultation in Pediatric Neurology: 49 Clinical Questions* (pp 215-222).
© 2016 Taylor & Francis Group.

Table 41-1

Clues to Localization of Ataxia

	Cerebellum	Vestibular	Sensory
Ear problems (tinnitus, ear pain)	−	++	−
Nausea	±	++	−
Paresthesias or back pain	−	−	+
Mental status	Variable	Normal	Normal
Nystagmus	Common (unprovoked, not fatigable)	Sometimes (may be provoked by change in head position)	Rare
Muscle weakness	−	−	Often
Reflexes	Variable	Normal	↓↓ (in peripheral neuropathy)
Special exam findings	Trunk titubation while sitting	Positive Dix-Hallpike test	Positive Romberg

cerebellar syndromes present with prominent gait ataxia, and are seen in postinfectious cerebellitis, drug ingestions, and most inherited cerebellar syndromes.

Cerebellar hemispheric syndromes are seen with lesions to one or both cerebellar hemispheres and present with dysmetria, past pointing, limb clumsiness, and difficulty with rapid alternating movements, but not titubation (difficulty maintaining sitting posture). These are less common and should prompt consideration of mass lesions, stroke, or demyelinating disorders. Thus, imaging (brain magnetic resonance imaging [MRI]) should generally be performed with these syndromes. Isolated flocculonodular syndromes presenting with nystagmus alone are rare, but the flocculonodulus is involved in pan-cerebellar syndromes, which affect the entire cerebellum.

Causes of Ataxia

For an overview of the most common causes of ataxia by time course, see Table 41-2. A description of the most common causes is presented below.

TOXIC INGESTION/EXPOSURE

This is the most common cause of acute ataxia in adolescents, and the second most common cause in all age groups.

Table 41-2
Most Common Causes of Ataxia by Time Course

Acute	*Recurrent*	*Acute or Chronic*
Toxic ingestion	Migraine/BPV	Tumor
ACA/postinfectious cerebellitis	Epileptic ataxia	Congenital malformations
GBS (especially Miller-Fisher variant)	OMAS	Metabolic disorders
Acute disseminated encephalomyelitis	Episodic ataxias	OMAS
Cerebellar stroke	Metabolic/mitochondrial disorders	
Trauma	Multiple sclerosis	
Labyrinthitis	Hypoglycemia	
Hypoglycemia	Antiphospholipid antibody syndrome	
OMAS		
Infectious encephalitis		

BPV: benign paroxysmal vertigo of childhood; ACA: acute cerebellar ataxia; GBS: Guillain-Barré syndrome; OMAS: opsoclonus-myoclonus-ataxia syndrome.

PRESENTATION

Accidental ingestions take place most commonly between ages 1 to 4, while intentional ingestions take place more often in adolescents. Clues to a toxic ingestion include altered mental status, inappropriate behavior, and prominent vomiting. Time course is often maximal at onset, although with some delayed-released drugs or drugs with a long half-life there may continue to be progression of symptoms over hours.

ETIOLOGY

The most common ingestions vary by the age of the child, their environment, and the substances available to them. A list of the most common toxins is found in Table 41-3.

TREATMENT

Treatment will vary by ingestion, and contact with a poison control center is generally recommended.

	Table 41-3	
Common Drugs/Toxins Causing Acute Ataxia		
Environmental Toxins	*Drugs: Younger Children*	*Drugs: Adolescents*
Lead	Anticonvulsants (especially phenytoin, carbamazepine, phenobarbital, benzodiazepines)	Alcohol
Carbon monoxide	Anticholinergics (especially found in over-the-counter cold medicines)	Drugs of abuse (especially marijuana, PCP, GHB, Robitussin [guaifenesin], opioids, solvents)
Cyanide	Oral hypoglycemics	Antidepressants
Insecticides	Cardiac medications (especially clonidine)	Antipsychotics
PCP: phencyclidine; GHB: gamma hydroxybutyrate.		

POSTINFECTIOUS ACUTE CEREBELLAR ATAXIA/ POSTINFECTIOUS CEREBELLITIS

These entities likely represent a spectrum of disorders in which a response to an infection or vaccination triggers an autoimmune attack on the cerebellum. It is often referred to as acute cerebellar ataxia (ACA) when imaging is normal and the presentation is relatively mild, and post-infectious cerebellitis when imaging shows inflammation of the cerebellum or the presentation is more severe, but there is no clear pathophysiologic difference between these disorders.

PRESENTATION

This typically occurs in children ages 2 to 5 with a pan-cerebellar or midline cerebellar syndrome (ie, prominent gait ataxia and instability of posture) occurring anywhere from 3 to 30 days after an infection or vaccination. Ataxia is usually maximal at onset and begins to improve after 2 to 3 days. Children are usually well appearing, have normal mental status, and are not profoundly irritable or uncomfortable. Cranial nerve exam should be normal aside from nystagmus.

ETIOLOGY

The most common infection reported in association with ACA is varicella, but Epstein-Barr virus (EBV), human herpesvirus 6 (HHV6), and multiple other viruses, bacterial infections, and vaccination exposures have been reported. Identifying a specific virus is often impossible and rarely helpful.

DIAGNOSIS

This is a clinical diagnosis. MRI is usually normal but may show T2 hyperintense signal and contrast enhancement of the cerebellum. Extracerebellar findings should prompt an alternative diagnosis such as acute disseminated encephalomyelitis (see below). Lumbar puncture is usually normal and therefore unnecessary unless an alternative diagnosis is suspected. Lumbar puncture may show a lymphocytic pleocytosis or an elevation of protein concentration.

TREATMENT

Treatment is supportive. Early consultation with physical therapy may be helpful to prevent falls. Case reports and small series have described treatment with steroids, intravenous immuno-globulin (IVIG), and other immunomodulatory therapy in severe or refractory cases, but there is no evidence for their effectiveness, and outcomes are good without treatment in most cases.

PROGNOSIS

Ninety percent of patients will be nearly fully recovered within 1 month, with 90% of the remaining patients functionally recovered by 1 year. Older age and preceding infection with EBV may be associated with worse prognosis. Failure to improve within 1 month of presentation should prompt consideration of alternative diagnoses, especially opsoclonus-myoclonus-ataxia syndrome (OMAS), and further evaluation and imaging should be performed. Recurrence is rare and should prompt consideration of alternative diagnoses (see Table 41-2 for causes of recurrent ataxia).

BENIGN PAROXYSMAL VERTIGO OF CHILDHOOD

Thought to be a migraine variant, this typically presents in children ages 3 to 5 with recurrent episodes of vertigo and ataxia lasting minutes to hours, often associated with vomiting, nausea, and autonomic changes such as pallor or sweating. It is sometimes, though certainly not always, accompanied by migraine headache, and patients sometimes evolve to having more typical migraines as they get older. Clues to the diagnosis include recurrent stereotyped episodes of vestibular ataxia with a complete return to normal (usually within several hours) and a family history of migraine. Prophylactic treatment is usually unnecessary unless episodes are frequent, in which case typical migraine medications such as cyproheptadine or topiramate may be useful.

GUILLAIN-BARRÉ SYNDROME

PRESENTATION

Guillain-Barré syndrome often presents with back pain and tingling in the hands and feet, followed by difficulty walking, while the Miller-Fisher variant of Guillain-Barré syndrome presents with ataxia, ophthalmoplegia, and areflexia. While the textbooks describe "ascending weakness" (or "length dependent weakness," referring to the length of the nerves involved), this is rarely apparent in younger children on presentation, who often simply look unsteady on their feet. Depressed deep tendon reflexes and lower extremity weakness are hallmarks of the disorder and should be apparent on detailed testing, however.

DIAGNOSIS

This is a clinical diagnosis. Lumbar puncture showing high protein with normal cells can be helpful, but at initial presentation cerebrospinal fluid (CSF) can be normal, with protein often taking days to rise. Conversely, a very high CSF protein (> 250 mg/dL) at presentation should direct the clinician to look for other diagnoses (Chiari or mass blocking CSF flow). Nerve conduction studies can be confirmatory but these are rarely available on demand and treatment should not be delayed while waiting for confirmatory tests.

TREATMENT

IVIG or plasmapheresis should be administered as soon as possible to prevent progression. IVIG is preferred at our center because of its rapid availability and the difficulties of placing pheresis catheters in small children. Respiratory reserve should be monitored carefully and a net inspiratory force should be obtained at presentation and then at regular intervals to trend function. Physical therapy can be helpful once patients have stabilized.

CONCUSSION/TRAUMA

While this is usually obvious in older children and adolescents, younger children who have been the victim of nonaccidental trauma may present solely with ataxia.

CEREBELLAR STROKE

This is a relatively uncommon cause of ataxia in healthy children, but should be considered in patients with asymmetric symptoms (worse on one side of the body) or with hypercoagulable states (eg, sickle cell disease, oncology patients), heart disease, recent head or neck trauma, or patients who are not following a typical time course for recovery. Presentation can be identical to that for ACA but the ataxia is more likely to be unilateral. Cerebellar swelling after stroke can be a life-threatening emergency leading to brainstem herniation; if the diagnosis is suspected, urgent imaging is recommended. Workup and management of stroke are detailed in Questions 33 and 36.

ACUTE DISSEMINATED ENCEPHALOMYELITIS

Acute disseminated encephalomyelitis is an acute demyelinating disorder that may present with acute ataxia, but ataxia is always accompanied by change in mental status or seizures. If suspected, acute imaging is required as this is potentially a life-threatening emergency. Treatment is with high-dose steroids and/or IVIG.

OPSOCLONUS-MYOCLONUS-ATAXIA SYNDROME

While this is an uncommon disorder overall, it should always be considered in patients who present with suspected ACA who fail to return to baseline within the expected time course. This disorder classically presents in younger children (typical age range 2 to 5 years) with ataxia, abnormal eye movements ("dancing eyes"), and myoclonic jerks ("dancing feet/hands"), but it may present with ataxia alone. Clues to the diagnosis include profound irritability, ataxia that is progressive rather than maximal at onset, and developmental regression. This may be a paraneoplastic syndrome and thus a thorough evaluation for neuroblastoma is required.

NON-NEUROLOGIC CAUSES OF ATAXIA (EG, CONVERSION DISORDER/PSYCHOGENIC ATAXIA)

Look for "astasia-abasia," an exaggerated inability to stand upright with lots of upper body movement but relatively narrow-based gait, as though the patient were pretending to walk on an imaginary tightrope. If this is suspected, an evaluation for abuse should always be conducted. (See Question 43 for more information.)

Evaluation

KEY ELEMENTS OF THE HISTORY

- Exact time course
  - When did the symptoms start? Were they maximal at onset or did they progress over time? Has the child improved at all over the last few hours, is he or she stable, or getting worse? Did the child have any problems with balance before this started? Has anything like this happened before?
- Medications or other substances
  - Parents should always be asked for a complete list of all medications and other drugs in the house and taken by family members.
- Recent illnesses or vaccinations
- Any possibility of trauma
- Family history of ataxia, migraine, seizures, or other neurologic disorders
- Associated symptoms
  - Ask about irritability, excessive sleepiness, change in hearing or ear pain, back pain, vomiting, abdominal pain, paresthesias, visual changes, and headaches.

LABS AND IMAGING

- Toxicology screening labs should be performed in almost all children with ACA. Anticonvulsants, antihypertensives, and antihistamines are common exposures in younger children whereas alcohol and drugs of abuse should be evaluated in adolescents. A serum glucose should be checked in younger children to check for oral hypoglycemic ingestion and metabolic causes of hypoglycemia.
- Head imaging: MRI of the brain should be performed if a clear etiology is not apparent from the history and physical exam. Though not evidence based, it is our practice to conduct an MRI with and without contrast in all patients with ACA for whom a drug exposure is unlikely and who have an atypical clinical picture for postinfectious cerebellitis. Computed tomography (CT) scans are rarely helpful as they image the cerebellum poorly; the exception is in the very ill child in whom impending herniation must be ruled out.
- Lumbar puncture can be reserved for those patients who are ill appearing, febrile, or otherwise have atypical presentations. Postinfectious cerebellitis may have a normal CSF profile or may have a mild lymphocytic pleocytosis. This is typically in the range of 10 to 20 white blood cell (WBC) count; a WBC count much higher than this, left shift, very high protein, or high red blood cell (RBC) count is generally suggestive of an alternative diagnosis, though some cases of postinfectious cerebellitis have had CSF WBC counts over 100.
- If OMAS is suspected, it is my practice to send urine catecholamines (homovanillic acid [HVA]/vanillylmandelic acid [VMA], spot or 24-hour collection) as well as obtaining a whole-body MRI scan, whole-body CT with contrast or iodine-131-meta-iodobenzylguanidine (MIBG) scintiscan looking for neuroblastoma. Note that the sensitivity of HVA/VMA is low and thus this test by itself is not enough to rule out neuroblastoma.

- In a critically ill child, an arterial blood gas sample may give clues regarding metabolic disorders. Additional metabolic testing such as lactate/pyruvate, urine organic acids, serum amino acids, and acylcarnitine profile may be recommended in consultation with a neurologist but is rarely sent on a first-pass evaluation.
- Other labs such as complete blood count, electrolytes, inflammatory markers, and liver function tests are rarely helpful except in critically ill children.

Suggested Readings

Fogel BL. Childhood cerebellar ataxia. *J Child Neurol.* 2012;27(9):1138-1145.

Gieron-Korthals MA, Westberry KR, Emmanuel PJ. Acute childhood ataxia: 10-year experience. *J Child Neurol.* 1994;9(4):381-384.

Ryan MM, Engle EC. Acute ataxia in childhood. *J Child Neurol.* 2003;18(5):309-316.

Salas AA, Nava A. Acute cerebellar ataxia in childhood: initial approach in the emergency department. *Emerg Med J.* 2010;27(12):956-957.

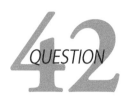

How Do You Distinguish Weakness From Ataxia?

Amy T. Waldman, MD, MSCE

Abnormal motor function is caused by a variety of neurologic disorders ranging from upper motor neuron lesions in the central nervous system to peripheral muscle disease. The localization of motor disturbances may be difficult, especially in differentiating weakness from ataxia in some patients. However, this distinction will inform upon the differential diagnosis and necessary evaluation and requires a careful neurologic examination.

Weakness is defined as the decreased ability of the muscles to generate force for voluntary movement against gravity and resistance. In order to separate weakness, or decreased muscle power, from cerebellar pathology, it is critical to understand the primary function of the cerebellum. The cerebellum coordinates motor movements by integrating sensory and other input from the spinal cord and brainstem. Therefore, cerebellar disease or injury results in difficulty with motor control and smooth movements. Of note, the cerebellum also plays a role in motor planning, cognition, and affective and autonomic function.

The most notable symptom localizing to the cerebellum is ataxia, which is broadly defined as the disturbance in the smooth performance of voluntary movement. The term *ataxia* is often used to describe an abnormal gait (gait ataxia) although cerebellar disease may also cause limb ataxia or truncal ataxia. Sensory ataxia is caused by damage to the proprioceptive (knowledge of position in space) pathways providing input to the cerebellum.

Before assessing cerebellar function, the motor examination is typically performed to assess bulk, tone, and strength. The patient's muscles are inspected for atrophy or asymmetry. Muscle atrophy occurs in various disorders but is not a feature of cerebellar disease. The patient's position should also be noted. Weakness may result in an externally rotated leg while lying down or a depressed shoulder while sitting. Next, tone is assessed in a relaxed patient by passively moving the muscles. Hypotonia, while not a prominent feature of cerebellar disease, can be seen after acute cerebellar injury or with chronic cerebellar disorders. Acutely, upper motor neuron disease in the

Licht DJ, Ryan NR, eds. *Curbside Consultation in Pediatric Neurology: 49 Clinical Questions* (pp 223-229).
© 2016 Taylor & Francis Group.

brain or spinal cord may cause hypotonia; however, such lesions ultimately result in spasticity or increased tone. Basal ganglia disease results in hypertonia or rigidity.

Next, muscle strength is assessed through confrontational muscle testing (Table 42-1). The examiner should attempt to isolate the muscle or muscle groups being tested, using one hand to support the limb while using the other hand to provide resistance. Conventionally, upper limb muscles are evaluated while sitting, and lower extremity muscles are evaluated while the patient is lying down. In the cooperative patient, strength should be checked in various positions (such as sitting and lying supine to test lower extremity function).

For children too young to participate in formal strength testing, gross testing can be performed, at the very least demonstrating antigravity movement, and the following functional tests may be informative. Upper extremity weakness can be detected in younger children (10 months and older) through the parachute reflex. While holding the child, the upper torso is moved forward so that the child has to place both hands in front of the body to protect the face. Asymmetric placement of the hands is abnormal, suggesting weakness or tone asymmetry of the hand that is not used. Subtle weakness in older children can be assessed by having the child assume a "wheelbarrow" position. Holding the child's feet, have the child "walk" on his or her hands. The pronator drift detects upper extremity weakness due to an upper motor neuron lesion: both arms are extended in front of the body with the palms facing upward. The patient is asked to hold the position with the eyes closed. Slight downward and internal rotation (pronation) of the forearm or curling of the fingers is abnormal.

Lower extremity strength can be assessed by asking the child to stoop (squat) and recover. Children should also be instructed to quickly rise from lying down. Children with muscular dystrophy are unable to rise quickly because of proximal (hip/shoulder girdle) weakness. These children need to "walk" their hands up the legs to stand (called Gowers' maneuver). Asking the child to walk on his or her toes and heels is another way to assess dorsiflexion and plantarflexion of the foot and ankle and distal leg function (see Table 42-1).

Cerebellar testing often begins with the patient seated to evaluate truncal and limb ataxia. Truncal ataxia occurs with midline cerebellar disease and causes an inability to sit or stand without support because of instability in postural musculature. There are a number of tests that can be performed to evaluate limb ataxia. The finger-to-nose test is used to evaluate dysmetria or intention tremor. Dysmetria occurs when the fingertip misses the target whereas intention tremor is characterized by oscillations of the limb upon reaching the target. Typically, intention tremor from cerebellar disease affects the proximal muscles causing fluctuations in amplitude of the limb. In contrast, essential tremor involves movement of the distal limbs only.

Limb ataxia can also manifest as an action tremor or impaired rapid alternating movements (called dysdiadochokinesis). To assess for an action tremor, the patient should extend his or her arms in front of the body or point the tips of his or her index fingers at each other without touching. Rapid alternating movements, such as supinating and pronating the hand, are irregular in cerebellar disease.

The ataxic gait is wide based (with the feet spread apart) and characterized by irregular or uncoordinated steps. Balance is impaired, often causing the patient to fall or stagger. Patients with unilateral cerebellar disease will fall to the ipsilateral side (or to the side of the lesion). Subtle difficulties are magnified by asking the patient to walk a straight line (tandem gait). Patients with gait ataxia cannot perform a tandem gait, with one foot directly placed in front of the other foot, or they will fall.

Additional clues from the neurologic examination can be used to further determine whether a cerebellar process is present. Other signs and symptoms of cerebellar disease include eye movement disorders and speech abnormalities. The most commonly noted eye movement disorder is nystagmus, in which there is an irregular oscillation of the eyes. Nystagmus is often characterized by a fast phase and a slow phase; the quick phase as the eyes are directed toward an object and the

Table 42-1

Distinguishing Weakness From Ataxia:
The Neurologic Examination and Localization of Deficits

Symptom/Sign	Test	Instructions	Abnormal Findings	Localization
Weakness (Can Be Caused by Many Disorders)				
Weakness	Muscle strength	Assess each muscle individually for spontaneous movement, against gravity, and against resistance and compare it to the muscle on the opposite side of the body	Scored on a scale of 0 to 5 as follows: 0/5: No contraction or movement of the muscle 1/5: Flicker of movement 2/5: Movement but not against gravity 3/5: Movement against gravity but not against resistance 4/5: Movement against gravity and some resistance 5/5: Full strength	Upper or lower motor neuron lesions
	Functional tests	Assess the symmetry and ability of children through different maneuvers such as quickly rising from a lying down position	When rising from a supine position, children have to use their hands to "climb" up their legs (Gowers' maneuver)	Disorder of muscle
		Ask the child to rise from a seated position and/or squat and recover	Proximal weakness	Upper or lower motor neuron lesion or disorder of muscle, neuromuscular junction, or nerve

(continued)

Table 42-1 (continued)

Distinguishing Weakness From Ataxia:
The Neurologic Examination and Localization of Deficits

Symptom/Sign	Test	Instructions	Abnormal Findings	Localization
		Ask the child to wheelbarrow (walk on the hands)	Proximal weakness	Upper or lower motor neuron lesion or disorder of muscle, neuromuscular junction, or nerve
	Pronator drift	Ask the patient to extend the arms in front of him or her with the palms facing up and close the eyes	The patient is unable to maintain the posture as the arm drifts downward and pronates (rotates inward)	Upper or lower motor neuron lesion or disorder of muscle, neuromuscular junction, or nerve
Tone	Passive range of motion	Passively move the arms and legs	Hypertonia (increased tone) or hypotonia (decreased tone)	Hypertonia (upper motor neuron lesion) or hypotonia (lower motor neuron lesion or cerebellar disease)
Bulk	Visual assessment of muscle size	Inspect and compare the size of the muscles on the left and right sides of the body	Atrophy	Lower motor neuron lesion

(continued)

Table 42-1 (continued)

Distinguishing Weakness From Ataxia:
The Neurologic Examination and Localization of Deficits

Symptom/Sign	Test	Instructions	Abnormal Findings	Localization
Cerebellar Disease				
Truncal ataxia	Gait	Walk across the room or down a hallway	Wide based (feet are wide to maintain balance)	Cerebellar vermis (midline lesions) or bilateral cerebellar lesions or unilateral lesions (patients fall to the side of the lesion)
	Posture	Ask the patient to sit without support	Difficulty sitting up without support	
	Tandem gait	Walk in a straight line while touching the heel to toe	Unable to maintain balance and posture	
Appendicular ataxia	Finger-nose-finger	Touch the examiner's finger, then his or her nose and back to the finger	Dysmetria (overshoot or undershoot the target, also called past-pointing)	Intermediate and lateral portions of the cerebellum (the lesion is ipsilateral or on the same side of the abnormal extremity)
	Heel-to-shin	Touch the knee with the opposite heel, slide the heel down the shin and back up	Difficulty with smooth movements up and down the shin	
	Rapid alternating movements	Pronation and supination of the hand (tap one palm on the other and then turn the hand over to touch the dorsum of the hand to the palm of the hand) or have the patient tap the hand or foot rapidly or touch the finger and thumb repeatedly	Dysdiadochokinesia (abnormal rhythm of movements)	

(continued)

Table 42-1 (continued)

Distinguishing Weakness From Ataxia:
The Neurologic Examination and Localization of Deficits

Symptom/Sign	Test	Instructions	Abnormal Findings	Localization
Eye movements	Cranial nerves (covered elsewhere), saccades, and pursuit	Ask the patient to follow the examiner's finger with his or her eyes in all directions (pursuit or slow conjugate eye movements)	Eye movements are not smooth and jerk or jump from side to side	Brainstem (covered elsewhere) and cerebellar vermis and flocculonodular lobes (midline lesions)
		The patient rapidly looks from one target to another target, such as the examiner's fingers held on either side of the face or a finger in the periphery to a midline target such as the examiner's nose (saccades or fast conjugate eye movements)	Ocular dysmetria (the eyes overshoot the target)	
		Eye movements, pursuit, and saccades	Vertical or direction-changing nystagmus	

slow phase occurs as the eyes drift back toward the neutral position. Smooth pursuit of the eyes is tested by having the patient follow the examiner's finger as it is moved in all directions. To assess saccades, the patient quickly looks at something in the midline (such as the examiner's nose) and then an object in the periphery (the examiner's finger). In cerebellar disease, speech is irregular and slow, often with poor articulation and variable breathing, tone, and pitch.

The differential diagnosis for weakness and ataxia is dependent on the involved muscles or body parts and time course. For example, acute unilateral weakness of a limb occurs in ischemic or hemorrhage stroke or spinal cord compression whereas episodic or chronic diffuse muscle weakness is seen in disorders of the neuromuscular junction and muscle. Acute gait ataxia in children typically follows an infection, ingestion, or drug toxicity whereas episodic or chronic ataxia occurs in hereditary ataxia and metabolic disease. A detailed neurologic examination and careful consideration of the localization of abnormal findings will aid in differentiating weakness from ataxia.

Suggested Readings

Liu GT, Volpe NJ, Galetta SL. *Neuro-Ophthalmology: Diagnosis and Management.* 2nd ed. Philadelphia, PA: Saunders Elsevier; 2010:551-586.

Maricich SM, Zoghbi HY. The cerebellum and the hereditary ataxias. In: Swaiman KF, Ashwal S, Ferriero DM, eds. *Pediatric Neurology: Principles and Practice.* 4th ed. Philadelphia, PA: Mosby Elsevier; 2006:1241-1269.

Sanger TD, Chen D, Delgado MR, et al. Definition and classification of negative motor signs in childhood. *Pediatrics.* 2006;118(5):2159-2167.

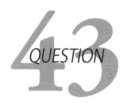

43

How Do You Tell a Pathologic Gait from a Functional Gait?

Laura A. Adang, MD, PhD

As neurologists, we are often asked to evaluate children with difficulty walking. The causes of an abnormal gait are extensive, but fall into nonexclusive general categories: neurologic, orthopedic, infectious, and other. In the literature, several interchangeable terms describe an abnormal gait without an organic cause, including hysterical, functional, and psychogenic. Astasia abasia (astasia = inability to stand upright, abasia = lack of motor coordination in walking) is the complete inability to walk without a physiologic cause. Other specific variations include functional camptocormia, which is walking with severe flexion at the waist. It is most common, however, for a functional gait disorder to include a variety of abnormal movements or deficits that are unexplainable by specific lesions in the nervous system. This chapter will attempt to help the reader distinguish functional gait disorder from true ataxias.

Psychogenic gaits are very common in pediatrics and more common in girls and have a mean age of onset of 12 years.[1] It is rare to have a psychogenic gait appear before the age of 10, although it has been reported in patients as young as 7 years old. These abnormal walking styles can involve a variety of abnormal movements that look like dystonia or chorea. Psychogenic gaits characteristically have an abrupt start and are often triggered by either a minor injury, like a fall, or a stressful event, such as bullying or a divorce in the family. The majority of children with psychogenic gaits are ultimately diagnosed with conversion disorder, which is an unconscious manifestation of a psychological stressor in a physical way, as opposed to malingering, which is more common in adults. Of note, most children do not have a pre-existing psychiatric history, and a triggering stressful event is not always identified.

There is a significant overlap between organic neurologic problems and functional movement disorders—between 10% and 40% of patients have both.[1] Patients will also elaborate on their neurologic symptoms to convince observers that the symptoms truly exist. When it is impossible to differentiate between a functional and organic gait disorder by history and physical examination,

Licht DJ, Ryan NR, eds. *Curbside Consultation in Pediatric Neurology: 49 Clinical Questions* (pp 231-234).
© 2016 Taylor & Francis Group.

a more extensive evaluation, often including imaging (such as magnetic resonance imaging of the brain or spine), electromyography, and laboratory testing, is warranted. Because of the fear on the part of the provider and the family of missing an underlying organic cause, it can take weeks to years to ultimately diagnose a functional gait disorder.

The neurologic physical exam, involving careful direct and indirect observation, can be particularly helpful in answering the question: Is this gait neurologic? First, it is important to watch the patient. Observe as he or she walks into and out of the clinic room, takes off his or her jacket, and climbs on the table. Often these routine movements reveal a lot about true motor strength and a possible underlying movement disorder. Watch the patient for motor inconsistency during the entire examination: Is he unable to perform rapid finger movements, but still able to text? Is she unable to walk during observation, but able to jump down quickly from the exam table? Beyond the standard gait assessment of walking, patients can be asked to walk in a straight line like on a tightrope, on the toes, on the heels, with eyes closed, and up and down a set of stairs. Each test gives additional information about proximal and distal strength, balance, and proprioception.

Specific testing during the examination of functional disorders can also be helpful. The Hoover sign can test for false weakness in the legs. There is a natural extension of the hip while attempting to flex on the other side, and therefore, with any attempted effort to lift our legs, we push down with the heel of our other leg. To perform, place your hand under the "good heel" and ask the patient to lift the weak leg and then alternate sides. Of note, if there is significant pain with movement, then the patient will not attempt to lift his or her leg, and thus the Hoover sign is unhelpful. The chair test can be performed by asking patients to propel themselves across the floor in a wheeled desk chair. Compare this demonstration of strength to that found on confrontation and gait testing. It is important to search for inconsistencies by testing the same muscle groups through a variety of direct and indirect tests. For example, casual observation of the patient rising from the chair can be compared to direct confrontation testing of lifting the leg at the hip.

Nonorganic weakness can have a characteristic "collapsing weakness," in which the limb folds immediately to light touch, but normal strength is found during confrontation testing. Often patients require enthusiastic encouragement to give full effort, which typically improves "give-way" weakness. It can also be helpful to give explicit instructions, such as "At the count of 3, push as hard as you can against me." Sometimes the weakness that we perceive as clinicians reflects only a difficulty understanding our foreign and confusing instructions.

Neurologically abnormal gaits are the by-product of a real deficit and, therefore, fall into established categories. For example, a foot drop essentially causes an abnormal lengthening of the leg. There are only a finite number of ways to move your dropped foot to its forward target during a step. Circumduction brings the foot around in a circular pattern, while steppage raises the knee up higher to keep the foot from dragging. Functional gaits by definition do not have a neurologic cause, and therefore are more variable and change from moment to moment. The broad categories of functional gait disorders include dragging, fluctuating, slow, "walking on ice," psychogenic Romberg, noneconomic, and knee buckling (Table 43-1).[2,3] In general, a functional gait will not result in self-injury or serious falls. Exaggerated swaying or side steps without falling are warning signs that the gait is primarily non-neurologic.

Again, it is important to remember that many patients will elaborate on their neurologic symptoms to convince the clinician of the symptoms' seriousness. Also, some movement disorders can look like functional disorders because of their peculiar presentations. A rare disorder, such as paroxysmal kinesiogenic dyskinesia, can be misdiagnosed for years as functional. This disease is a problem of sudden abnormal movements, including choreoathetosis, dystonia, or ballismus, in one or several limbs that are triggered by sudden movements. Other neurologic diseases such as myasthenia gravis can fluctuate rapidly. Pain can also limit the speed of movements and the effort

Table 43-1
Common Types of Functional Gait Disorders

Type of Functional Gait	Description	Helpful Hints
Dragging monoplegic gait	A dragging limb during walking instead of circumduction	Confrontational testing for strength assessment and Hoover sign
Fluctuating gait	Distractible abnormalities	Finger-to-nose testing while standing
Slow or hesitant gait	Persistently slow movements or difficulty initiating steps	Distraction, assessment while texting if hands also affected
Psychogenic Romberg	Falls in predictable direction (typically toward or away from examiner), often accompanied by large swaying movements	Improves with distraction, examiner should change position to test directionality of falling
"Walking on ice" gait	Similar to someone walking on a slippery surface, such as ice, with broad-based steps that are small and stiff	No other signs of ataxia
Noneconomic posture	Involves excessive movements that are not to compensate for a neurologic deficits and are difficult to replicate because of the strength needed, such as walking crouched over	Improves with distraction
Knee buckling	Sudden loss of leg tone, but without falling or self-injury	Strength testing will be normal

given during an examination. As always, careful history and physical examination should aid in the proper diagnosis and the differentiation between functional and neurological symptoms. Patients with conversion disorders benefit from intensive therapies (physical and psychological) and rehabilitation, and the earlier they receive treatment, the better the long-term outcome. It is possible for a patient to develop severe contractures or other complications from persistent abnormal positioning with a functional gait disorder.

References

1. Schwingenschuh P, Pont-Sunyer C, Surtees R, Edwards M, Bhatia K. Psychogenic movement disorders in children: a report of 15 cases and a review of the literature. *Movement Disorders*. 2008;23:1882-1888.
2. Stone J, Zeman A, Sharpe M. Functional weakness and sensory disturbance. *J Neurol Neurosurg Psychiatry*. 2010;73(3):241-245.
3. Daum C, Hubschmid M, Aybek S. The value of positive clinical signs for weakness, sensory and gait disorders in conversion disorder: a systemic and narrative review. *J Neurol Neurosurg Psychiatry*. 2014;85(2):180-190.

SECTION XI

GENETIC

DEVELOPMENTAL DELAY

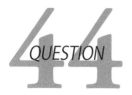

How Should I Begin a Workup for a Child With Significant Developmental Delay?

Ethan M. Goldberg, MD, PhD

The concept of global developmental delay (GDD) cannot meaningfully be extricated from that of intellectual disability; most patients with GDD are delayed in most or all developmental domains, including the cognitive domain. The question of how to address the workup for significant developmental delay necessitates a prior and proper diagnosis. The general pediatrician should be familiar with the tools used to assess childhood development. The diagnosis of developmental delay can be based on the results of appropriate psychometric or other testing or on expert judgment and extensive clinical experience.

The causes of significant developmental delay are vast, but are generally divided into 3 broad categories: prenatal/congenital (eg, chromosomal disorders and genetic/metabolic syndromes, in utero toxic or infectious exposures), perinatal (eg, hypoxic-ischemic brain injury, stroke), and postnatal/environmental (eg, lead poisoning, meningitis, head trauma) (Table 44-1). Many such causes can be readily diagnosed by the general pediatrician after a detailed history and physical examination, without further diagnostic testing. If the cause of the GDD is not readily apparent, then a medical workup should commence.

As mentioned, medical workup of a child with GDD (Figure 44-1) always includes a thorough history taking (including gestational, birth, and family history, with specific questions concerning possible in utero toxin exposures, prior pregnancy losses, parental consanguinity, etc), developmental assessment (including screening for autism spectrum disorder), and physical examination (with particular attention to growth parameters including head circumference, dysmorphology, congenital anomalies, neurocutaneous stigmata, and the neurologic exam). Referral to the specialist for ophthalmologic examination and/or audiometric evaluation can be useful at this point. Other questions to consider while performing the initial evaluation include: Is there a particular pattern of inheritance (eg, X-linked)? Are there specific associated abnormalities,

Licht DJ, Ryan NR, eds. *Curbside Consultation in Pediatric Neurology: 49 Clinical Questions* (pp 237-241). © 2016 Taylor & Francis Group.

Table 44-1

Common Causes of Significant Developmental Delay

Prenatal/Congenital

- Genetic
  - Single gene defects
  - Fragile X mental retardation syndrome
  - Tuberous sclerosis
  - Rett syndrome
  - Chromosomal abnormalities (deletions, duplications, aneuploidy, etc)
  - Trisomy 21
  - Prader-Willi syndrome
  - DiGeorge syndrome
  - 1p36 deletion syndrome
  - 15q11.2 deletion syndrome
  - 16p11.2 deletion/duplication syndrome
  - Metabolic (eg, phenylketonuria)
- Toxic exposures in utero (eg, fetal alcohol syndrome)
- Infectious (eg, TORCH infection)

Perinatal

- Extreme prematurity
- Hypoxia-ischemia
- Infectious (eg, herpes simplex virus, group B streptococcus meningoencephalitis)
- Neurovascular (eg, stroke, sinus venous thrombosis)

Postnatal/Environmental

- Environmental exposures (eg, lead)
- Neurovascular (eg, stroke)
- Nonaccidental trauma
- Inorganic causes
- Infectious

such as ophthalmologic (eg, cataracts), skin abnormalities (eg, ash leaf spots, café au lait macules), deafness, unexplained vomiting, hepatosplenomegaly, or short stature? It is important to note that diagnosis is best made over time rather than based on a single interaction, although certain red flags, such as seizures, developmental regression, and markedly increased or rapidly expanding head circumference, should prompt more urgent referral.

If the initial assessment does not suggest a specific diagnosis, the general practitioner should initiate further evaluation. However, it is useful at this point to consider whether developmental delay might be secondary to inorganic causes, another general medical condition or chronic illness, or another neuropsychiatric illness. The medical workup of significant developmental delay may further include genetic testing, metabolic/biochemical testing, neuroimaging (computed

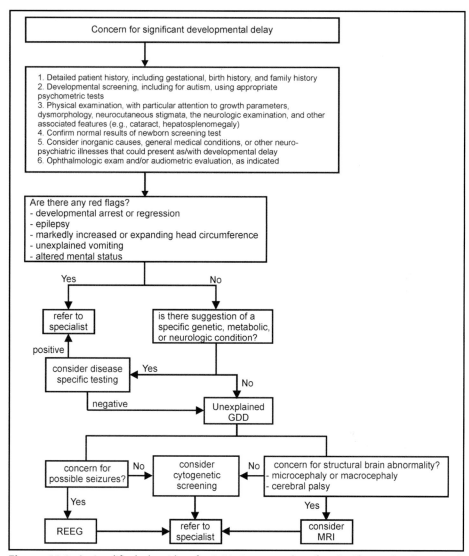

Figure 44-1. A simplified algorithm for initiating a workup for significant developmental delay. GDD: global developmental delay; MRI: magnetic resonance imaging; REEG: routine 20-minute electroencephalogram.

tomography and magnetic resonance imaging [MRI]), and electroencephalography, but should proceed in a stepwise fashion. The general pediatrician can initiate this medical workup by ordering first-tier tests in specific situations that are considered high yield and/or noninvasive. Second-tier testing should be deferred to the specialist. The American Academy of Neurology has published practice parameters on the evaluation of GDD and on the use of genetic and metabolic testing in the evaluation of GDD.

The utility of specific tests in the evaluation of significant developmental delay depends on a host of factors, including the cost and invasiveness of the test, the pretest probability of the test being positive based on the details of the case, and whether the results of testing will suggest a diagnosis that is treatable, among other considerations. Most decisions regarding genetic and metabolic testing are typically made by pediatric neurologists, medical geneticists, or specialists in metabolic disease.

Table 44-2
When to Refer the Patient With
Significant Developmental Delay to a Pediatric Neurologist

- Evaluation of unexplained global developmental delay
- Developmental arrest or regression
- Developmental delay "plus"[a]
- Result of initial testing (genetic or neuroimaging) is abnormal or of uncertain significance
- Syndromic autism[b]

[a]Accompanied by positive family history, micro- or macrocephaly, facial dysmorphism, congenital malformation, abnormal neurologic exam, autism spectrum disorder, history of unprovoked seizure or epilepsy.
[b]Autism plus dysmorphology, positive family history, abnormal neurologic examination, or epilepsy.

If there is a family history of GDD due to a known disorder, genetic or metabolic testing for that disease could be ordered. If there are specific features identified via history and physical examination to strongly suggest a specific disorder (such as Down syndrome, Fragile X syndrome, Rett syndrome, 22q11.2 deletion syndrome), then the appropriate specific diagnostic test can be ordered, based on the experience and level of comfort of the individual practitioner. For example, males with unexplained intellectual impairment and an X-linked pattern of inheritance may be screened for Fragile X syndrome; females with unexplained intellectual disability and characteristic repetitive hand movements may be screened for Rett syndrome. If there is a concern for seizure(s) or epilepsy, a routine electroencephalogram (EEG) could be ordered and the patient referred to a pediatric neurologist; it is useful to the neurologist if this EEG has been performed prior to the patient being seen in this situation. Otherwise, at this point, we recommend that the patient be referred to a pediatric neurologist (Table 44-2).

The genetic evaluation of a child with GDD for which a specific diagnosis is not immediately clear typically begins with genome-wide testing. This is most commonly a genome-wide microarray, which has replaced karyotyping and fluorescent in situ hybridization. We would consider array-based genome-wide testing a first-tier test for the general practitioner comfortable with its use. Microarray testing is diagnostic in approximately 7% to 8% of all cases of GDD, is considered to have the highest yield among genetic screening tests, and is accepted as the first-tier diagnostic test in the genetic workup of GDD or unexplained congenital anomalies. The yield increases in cases where the child has distinctive syndromic features or multiple congenital abnormalities. A major challenge in the use of array technology is the separation of the pathogenic from normal genetic variation; thus, the results of microarray testing may be ambiguous if not ordered in the proper context.

The reported yield of neuroimaging in the evaluation of significant developmental delay is variable, but is generally performed in parallel with first-tier genetic testing or if the results of a genome-wide microarray are normal or ambiguous. If performed for a specific indication, the yield is high. For example, it is appropriate for the primary care provider to order an MRI for the assessment of significant developmental delay in the patient with cerebral palsy. In children with cerebral palsy, a focal neurological exam, or epilepsy, an MRI of the brain may be the only test needed to yield an etiology for GDD.

Provided that standard newborn screening was performed and the results were normal, it is not indicated for the primary care provider to order metabolic screening tests for inborn errors of metabolism unless a specific disease is suggested by physical examination or family history.

Summary

The major role of the general pediatrician in the workup of significant developmental delay is in proper ascertainment and characterization of the delay, identification of red flags, if present, requiring urgent referral to the appropriate specialist, and initiation of the medical workup with first-tier testing as indicated based on the level of comfort and experience of the practitioner.

Suggested Readings

Michelson DJ, Shevell MI, Sherr EH, Moeschler JB, Gropman AL, Ashwal S. Evidence report: genetic and metabolic testing on children with global developmental delay: report of the Quality Standards Subcommittee of the American Academy of Neurology and the Practice Committee of the Child Neurology Society. *Neurology.* 2011;77(17):1629-1635.

Petersen MC, Kube DA, Palmer FB. Classification of developmental delays. *Semin Pediatr Neurol.* 1998;5(1):2-14.

Rosenberg SA, Zhang D, Robinson CC. Prevalence of developmental delays and participation in early intervention services for young children. *Pediatrics.* 2008;121(6):e1503-e1509.

Shevell M, Ashwal S, Donley D, et al. Practice parameter: evaluation of the child with global developmental delay: report of the Quality Standards Subcommittee of the American Academy of Neurology and the Practice Committee of the Child Neurology Society. *Neurology.* 2003;60(3):367-380.

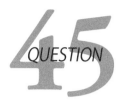

WHAT IS A GOOD APPROACH TO THINKING ABOUT A CHILD WITH MULTIPLE DYSMORPHISMS?

Mai T. Dang, MD, PhD

A dysmorphism is difference in a body structure. If the dysmorphia is truly the only abnormality that you see in the child, further evaluation is often unnecessary. Isolated dysmorphisms are typically caused by malformation (abnormal tissue development), deformation (distortion caused by a mechanic force), disruption (destruction of a normal forming structure), or dysplasia (anomaly of growth and differentiation). A patient with multiple dysmorphisms, however, typically requires further workup to arrive at the cause, which could be chromosomal, genetic, or environmental such as in utero exposure to teratogen or infection.[1] Making the diagnosis relies on recognizing the pattern of dysmorphisms. The 4 major patterns to consider are the following[2]:

1. Association: Physical features that often occur together more often than would be seen by chance alone, but no single etiology is yet known to explain the pattern. Vertebral anomalies, anal atresia, cardiac defects, trachea esophageal fistula, renal anomalies, and limb anomalies (VACTERL) are examples of associations with no unifying etiology.

2. Sequence: A group of defects that stem from a sequential set of events that began with one malformation. An example is Potter sequence with renal agenesis resulting in no fetal urine production, which leads to severe oligohydramnios with the consequences of lung hypoplasia and intrauterine constraint that cause limb deformities and compressed facial features.

3. Syndrome: A cluster of anomalies that occur in a consistent pattern that has a unifying cause, known or unknown.

4. Developmental field defect: A group of malformations caused by harm to a particular region of the embryo. An example is hemifacial microsomia, unilateral facial hypoplasia, and ear anomalies that come from anomalous development of the first and second brachial arch structures.

Licht DJ, Ryan NR, eds. *Curbside Consultation in Pediatric Neurology: 49 Clinical Questions* (pp 243-246). © 2016 Taylor & Francis Group.

When several obvious dysmorphisms are observed in a child, the evaluation should begin with the history and thorough physical examination to identify more subtle dysmorphisms. Special attention should be made to the following during the history and physical.[1-4]

History

PREGNANCY HISTORY

A child born extremely premature is at high risk of having cerebral palsy, vision and hearing problems, and long-term feeding and growth problems. Postmaturity could be a sign of trisomy 18 or anencephaly. Babies born after breech presentation have increased incidences of defects of form and/or function. Reduced fetal movements may themselves indicate a neuromuscular disorder. Exposure to teratogens such as alcohol and/or drugs and viruses could adversely affect the fetus. Small for gestational age may indicate chromosomal anomaly or result from teratogen exposure. Large for gestational age may be caused by a diabetic mother or an overgrowth syndrome such as Beckwith-Widemann syndrome.

PERINATAL HISTORY

Infant anthropometrics such as birth weight, length, and head circumference are important markers of growth. Some syndromes are associated with congenital microcephaly (present at birth) and others with acquired microcephaly (decreased growth velocity). Unexpectedly low Apgar scores in the absence of birth trauma are seen in neuromuscular disorders, Prader-Willi syndrome, or congenital myotonic dystrophy, among others.

FAMILY HISTORY

Health, developmental, or functional issues in the 3 generations starting from the patient need to be reviewed. A history of multiple miscarriages, stillbirth, death, and consanguinity should be noted.

Physical Examination

GROWTH

Height/length, weight, and head circumference and shape should be noted and plotted on appropriate growth curves. Special charts are available for certain disorders such as Down syndrome, Noonan syndrome, and achondroplasia. Note body proportions and asymmetry. Abnormal head shapes include dolichocephalic (long and thin), brachycephalic (short and wide), and plagiocephalic (asymmetric or lopsided).

FACIAL FEATURES

Look for asymmetry; sloping/deficiency or prominence of forehead; spacing of the eyes (hyper- or hypotelorism—far apart or too close, respectively) and slant (up or down) of the palpebral fissures (eyelid); shape and size of the nose tip or nares (nostrils), mouth, and chin; and size, shape, position, and orientation of the ears (low-set ears is defined as the upper edge of the ear falling below a line drawn from the inner canthus across the outer canthus to the occiput). Disorders of the palate such as clefting or high-arch palate can be seen in a number of syndromes including 22q- syndrome (DiGeorge, or velocardiofacial, syndrome).

NECK

Look for shortening that is seen in skeletal dysplasias and Klippel-Feil anomaly. Webbing is commonly seen in Turner and Noonan syndromes.

TRUNK

Auscultate the chest for any cardiac murmurs. Palpate the abdomen for organomegaly. Look at chest shape and spinal curvature. Shield-like chest is seen in Noonan and Turner syndromes. Pectus and scoliosis is seen in Marfan syndrome. Look at the back for the shape of the spine, sacral dimpling, hair tuft, and defects such as myelomeningocele.

EXTREMITIES

Look at the proportions of the limbs, muscle bulk and tone, joint contractures or webbing across large joints (pterygium), and mobility. Radioulnar synostosis occurs in fetal alcohol spectrum disorder and in some X chromosome aneuploidy (extra chromosomes) syndromes. Examine digits of the hand for the following: polydactyly (presence of extra digits seen in trisomy 13), oligodactyly (a deficiency in number of digits seen in Fanconi syndrome), brachydactyly (short fingers seen in Rubinstein Taybi syndrome), arachnodactyly (long, spidery fingers seen in Marfan syndrome or Soto syndrome), or syndactyly (joining of 2 or more digits, seen in many syndromes including Smith-Lemli-Opitz syndrome). Look at shape and length of digits, dermal ridges, and nails of hands and feet.

GENITALIA

Examine for abnormalities in structure. Ambiguous genitalia can be a sign of congenital adrenal hyperplasia and chromosomal disorders such as 45X/46XY.

Many sources are available to look up the set of dysmorphisms to arrive at a cause. They include the following:

- Textbooks of syndromes such as *Smith's Recognizable Patterns of Human Malformation.*
- Computerized databases where searches can be made using key dysmorphic features. Most of these require a subscription.
  - London Medical Database (www.lmdatabases.com/)
  - London Neurogenetics Database
  - Pictures of Standard Syndromes and Undiagnosed Malformations (POSSUM) (www.possum.net.au)

If a specific syndrome is suspected and a gene mutation is known to be the cause, genetic testing should be performed for confirmation. The comprehensive website www.genetest.org will direct you to the tests available for the suspected genetic disorder.

If a more general genetic evaluation is needed because no syndrome can yet be identified, the workup for a child with multiple dysmorphisms typically starts with a karyotype of blood lymphocytes to look for chromosomal rearrangement. Genome-wide array analysis is now widely available to identify large deletions or additions of DNA fragments and single-point mutations based on predetermined single nucleotide polymorphisms. Whole-exome sequencing provides the sequence for regions DNA that encodes all known proteins. This type of analysis is at this point the most comprehensive sequencing available for patients. However, it is expensive, takes several months, and often requires the expertise of a geneticist to interpret the results.

Depending on the syndrome, other common studies conducted for evaluation of multiple dysmorphisms include metabolic labs or imaging when applicable. Patients should be referred to a clinical geneticist, particularly when a diagnosis is challenging. Other specialists such as a neurologist may need to be consulted to help manage the complications of the syndrome.

References

1. Rimoin D, Korf BR. A clinical approach to the dysmorphic child. In: Rimoin DL, Pyeritz RE, Korf BR, eds. *Emery and Rimoin's Principle and Practice of Medical Genetics.* 6th ed. New York, NY: Elsevier; 2013.
2. South M, Isaacs D. The dysmorphic child. In: *Practical Paedatrics.* 7th ed. London, United Kingdom: Churchill Livingstone; 2012.
3. Gleason CA, Devaskar SU. Evaluation of the dysmorphic infant. In: *Avery's Diseases of the Newborn.* 9th ed. Philadelphia, PA: Elsevier/Saunders; 2012.
4. Marcdante KJ, Kliegman RM. The approach to the dysmorphic child. In: *Nelson Essentials of Pediatrics.* 7th ed. Philadelphia, PA: Elsevier/Saunders; 2014.

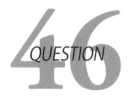

WHEN SHOULD I THINK ABOUT A MITOCHONDRIAL DISORDER, AND WHAT IS A GOOD APPROACH TO AN INITIAL EVALUATION?

Xilma R. Ortiz-Gonzalez, MD, PhD

Although our understanding of human genetics and bioenergetics continues to grow, clinically mitochondrial disorders remain challenging to diagnose and manage.[1] Mitochondria have their own circular DNA (mtDNA), which is maternally inherited, but beyond their traditionally taught role in generating energy via oxidative phosphorylation, they are also increasingly implicated in complex cellular functions including calcium homeostasis, apoptosis (programed cell death), and epigenetic regulation (regulation of gene expression in response to environmental cues) of nuclear genes.[2] Taking this into account, it is understandable that clinically mitochondrial dysfunction can present with progressive, multisystem disease.

If you are considering a mitochondrial disorder, a thorough history and exam are crucial, as there might be much heterogeneity in disease course and manifestations, even within the same family. A good place to start is eliciting a thorough medical history and in particular whether there is a history of neurodevelopmental regression. Neurologic decline, especially in the setting of fever or acute illness, is a red flag. It raises concern for metabolic disease, including, although by no means limited to, mitochondrial disease. A history of difficulty gaining weight or failure to thrive is consistent, although not always present. Careful review of systems with emphasis on vision, hearing, neurologic, and cardiac problems is key as well as a detailed family history for the same systems. Often undiagnosed progressive neurodegenerative complaints with onset in childhood or young adulthood are reported in the family history, such as progressive gait difficulties due to neuropathies or myopathy, optic neuropathies, white matter disease, atypical strokes, or dementia. The age of onset is often in young children, but it can range widely from neonates with cardiomyopathy to adults with optic atrophy. The inheritance pattern may be unclear, which can be confusing for providers and families. mtDNA-encoded genes exhibit inheritance along maternal lineage, but severity can fluctuate based on heteroplasmy levels (different amount of mutant mtDNA in different tissues). Also if the defect is present in a nuclear gene, Mendelian

Licht DJ, Ryan NR, eds. *Curbside Consultation in Pediatric Neurology: 49 Clinical Questions* (pp 247-251).
© 2016 Taylor & Francis Group.

Table 46-1
Possible Clinical Features of Mitochondrial Disorders

Organ System	Clinical Feature
Ophthalmological	Ptosis, optic nerve pallor or atrophy, ophthalmoplegia, pigmentary retinopathy, cataracts
Neurological	Ataxia, myopathy/weakness, exercise intolerance, peripheral neuropathy, epilepsy, myoclonus, dystonia, metabolic stroke, progressive encephalopathy
Renal	Renal tubular acidosis, generalized amino aciduria
Cardiac	Cardiomyopathy (hypertrophic or dilated), cardiac conduction defects
Ear, nose, and throat	Sensorineural hearing loss (including aminoglycoside induced)
Bone marrow	Sideroblastic anemia
Gastrointestinal	Elevated transaminases, gastrointestinal dysmotility, hepatopathy
Endocrine	Diabetes

transmission in dominant, recessive, or X-linked fashion is possible. A progressive disease course is highly suggestive of a metabolic disorder but keep in mind that in young children this is not always evident.

Although developmental delay, hypotonia, and/or seizures are frequently reported in mitochondrial disease, they are nonspecific and common to many neurodevelopmental disorders. Some of the common clinical features that will raise your suspicion of a mitochondrial cytopathy are listed in Table 46-1. Taken individually, none of these clinical features is specific for mitochondrial disorder, and unfortunately there is no single pathognomonic sign for the disease. Rather, the complete clinical picture, including clinical course, exam findings, and family history, needs to be taken into account.

A comprehensive physical exam is key and can be targeted toward finding evidence for the disease features listed in Table 46-1. For example, a funduscopic exam is very helpful to screen for optic atrophy or pigmentation abnormalities of the retina (salt and pepper retinopathy). A neurologic exam in search of features like ophthalmoplegia, ptosis, ataxia, weakness, or abnormal reflexes remains paramount in the evaluation.

Diagnostic evaluation has been traditionally based on biochemical serum markers (lactic acidosis, hyperalaninemia) or functional studies (electron transport chain [ETC] and respirometry assays in affected tissue, often liver or muscle biopsy specimen). Recently, this approach is largely complemented by genetic testing. Nevertheless, a baseline evaluation often includes the following.

Labs

Comprehensive metabolic panel, plasma and/or cerebrospinal fluid lactate levels, total and free carnitine levels, acylcarnitine profile, plasma amino acids, and urine organic acids.

Consults

Referral to ophthalmology, cardiology, and neurology is often considered to further evaluate for signs of mitochondrial disease.

Imaging

Brain magnetic resonance imaging with magnetic resonance spectroscopy is often helpful if neurologic symptoms are present.

Further evaluation and diagnostic testing are often performed by subspecialists in metabolism, genetics, or neurogenetics. Mutant mtDNA can exhibit heteroplasmy (different tissues may differ in mutant mtDNA amount and distribution); therefore, when possible, tissue samples from an involved/symptomatic organ is preferred for biochemical testing. Tissue samples can then be used to assay respiratory function (ETC activity) and mtDNA copy number, and evaluate for mtDNA point mutations or somatic deletions. Nomenclature can be confusing to families and providers as many mitochondrial disorders were initially described as clinical syndromes based on the phenotype, which have since then been proven to be caused by a multitude of genetic changes that result in mitochondrial dysfunction. As we gain further insight into the molecular causes of the syndromes and learn about new mutations that cause them, it is increasingly evident that there is significant overlap in their phenotypes. If the patient indeed fits a distinct clinical syndrome (Table 46-2), or a familial mutation is known, targeted genetic testing may be pursued. Most often, given the overlap of the phenotypes, next-generation sequencing panels are used to evaluate both for nuclear and mtDNA-encoded genes that are known to be associated with mitochondrial disease. Clinical judgment and biochemical findings remain pivotal as not all nuclear genes involved in mitochondrial function are well understood, limiting our current ability to confirm the diagnosis at a molecular level.

Treatment remains supportive, and although the intrinsic heterogeneity of mitochondrial diseases makes randomized clinical trials a challenge, as we gain further understanding of the extensive list of genes that underlie mitochondrial disorders, new strategies are being investigated.[3] Most often a mitochondrial cocktail of vitamins and supplements is prescribed with the rationale of supporting mitochondrial function. Although many of the supplements are available without prescription, it often facilitates compliance to prescribe a custom-compounded cocktail containing all the supplements for ease of administration. Typically the cocktail includes CoQ10 (as ubiquinol or ubiquinone), B-complex vitamins, vitamin C, vitamin E, folinic acid, L-creatine, L-carnitine, and alpha lipoic acid.[4]

Table 46-2

Some Clinical Syndromes Caused by Mitochondrial Dysfunction

Syndrome	Defining Features	Common Genes
MELAS	Mitochondrial encephalopathy, lactic acidosis, and stroke-like episodes	MT-TL1, MT-ND5
NARP	Neurogenic weakness, ataxia, retinitis, pigmentosa	MT-ATP6
MERRF	Myoclonic epilepsy with ragged ref fibers	MT-TK, MT-TF
MNGIE	Mitochondrial neurogastrointestinal encephalpmyopathy-PEO, leukoencephalopathy, neuropathy, GI dysmotility	TYMP, POLG
LHON	Leber's hereditary optic neuropathy: rapid monocular visual loss in one eye, later followed by the other eye, onset often late teens/young adult, more penetrant in males	MT-ND4, MT-ND6, MT-ND1, MT-ND2, MT-ND5, MT-CYB, MT-CO3
Alper's-Huttenlocher (mitochondrial-depletion syndromes)	Initially described as hepatocerebral disease with infantile onset of hypotonia, developmental regression, seizures, liver failures; but increasingly heterogeneous presentations including adults with neuropathy, myopathy, PEO, ptosis, progressive encephalopathy, sensory ataxia, dysarthria, cardiomyopathy	POLG, MVP17, DGUOK, RRM2B, SUCLA2, SUCLG1, TK2, C10ORF2
Leigh's	Subacute necrotizing relapsing encephalopathy with onset in infancy, developmental regression, seizures, brainstem and/or basal ganglia lesions, hepatopathy, movement disorder, decompensation with illness	Multiple mtDNA and nuclear genes, including MT-ATP6, MT-TL1, MT-ND1, MT-ND2, MT-ND3, MT-ND4, MT-ND5, MT-ND6; SURF1, NDUFS1, NDUFS4, LRPPRC
PEO[a]	Progressive external ophthalmoplegia, ± ptosis, mild proximal myopathy	ANT1, PEO1, POLG2
KSS[a]	Kearns-Sayre syndrome: PEO at age < 20 years, pigmentary retinopathy, ± cardiac conduction defects or ataxia	> 150 mtDNA deletions, m.8470_13446del4977 is the most common

(continued)

Table 46-2 (continued)
Some Clinical Syndromes Caused by Mitochondrial Dysfunction

Syndrome	Defining Features	Common Genes
Pearson[a]	Sideroblastic anemia/pancytopenia, exocrine pancreas failure (diabetes, malabsorption), renal tubular dysfunction	mtDNA deletions, detectable in leukocytes

[a]Also classified as mitochondrial deletion syndromes.

PEO: progressive external ophthalmoplegia; mtDNA: mitochondrial DNA.

References

1. Mitochondrial Medicine Society's Committee on Diagnosis, Haas RH, Parikh S, et al. The in-depth evaluation of suspected mitochondrial disease. *Mol Genet Metab.* 2008;94(1):16-37.
2. Wallace DC, Fan W. Energetics, epigenetics, mitochondrial genetics. *Mitochondrion.* 2010;10(1):12-31.
3. Koopman WJ, Willems PH, Smeitink JA. Monogenic mitochondrial disorders. *N Engl J Med.* 2012;366(12):1132-1141.
4. Parikh S, Saneto R, Falk MJ, et al. A modern approach to the treatment of mitochondrial disease. *Curr Treat Options Neurol.* 2009;11(6):414-430.

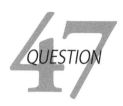

WHAT ARE THE NEURODEVELOPMENTAL DISORDERS LEADING TO LANGUAGE DELAY AND WHAT WORKUP IS NEEDED?

Laufey Yr Sigurdardottir, MD

Joey is a 3.5-year-old boy who presents for evaluation of developmental delay. His parents describe the following: Joey was a healthy infant who displayed normal motor development in the first year of life. He was walking independently at 12 months of age and had approximately 5 to 8 words at the age of 14 months. At the age of 18 months he went through a 2-week period of irritability and "being as if in his own world." He stopped acknowledging his parents' voices and started exhibiting peculiar behavior such as walking in circles and hitting his head repeatedly. Following this 2-week period, little Joey has been "a different child" with poor verbal skills, little interest in social interaction, and prominent self-stimulatory behavior.

Eli is also 3.5 years old and is brought into the office for developmental delay. His parents describe Eli as being a healthy infant who was "a little late taking off" with his motor abilities. Eli did not fixate on objects until 3 months of age, he did not hold toys until 7 months of age, and did not sit unsupported until 11 months of age. Eli started walking independently at 22 months of age and currently has a 20-word vocabulary. Eli enjoys the company of his parents and will pull, point, and grunt until they understand his wants. Eli enjoys playing with simple toys geared for toddlers and seems to need more time to learn new skills than his peers. He can be frustrated but is always interested in interacting with his parents and peers.

Joey and Eli are referred for a multidisciplinary evaluation, looking at their developmental quotient (verbal and nonverbal intelligence quotient), language development (receptive and expressive language quotients), adaptive behavior skills, fine and gross motor development, and for further evaluation of possible autistic features. It comes as no surprise that both of them have a neurodevelopmental disorder. Joey is found to have childhood autism while Eli is diagnosed with an intellectual disability. So what is the difference between the 2 boys? What are the possible neurodevelopmental disorders leading to speech delay in children?

There are 3 neurodevelopmental disorders that come to mind.

Licht DJ, Ryan NR, eds. *Curbside Consultation in Pediatric Neurology: 49 Clinical Questions* (pp 253-255).
© 2016 Taylor & Francis Group.

The first, specific language impairment, leads to prominent delays in expressive or expressive/receptive language while spatial, visual, and nonverbal skills and adaptive behavior remain within normal limits. These children may have behavioral difficulties but do not have poor social interaction or marked repetitive or peculiar behavior. They have poor speech development from an early age and do not have history of developmental stagnation or regression. These children have normal imitation, gesturing, and eye contact and are quick to pick up on visual cues. All children will benefit from speech therapy and some will function without special education services in elementary school, but the majority of children with specific language impairment need ongoing therapy and supportive services throughout early education.

The second, intellectual disability, leads to global delays in verbal and nonverbal development along with significant delays in adaptive behavior skills. These children will often have a history of delay in motor development followed by delays in speech development. They follow a slow upward developmental trajectory and periods of developmental regression are typically not seen. These children have social communication skills that are at the level of their overall cognitive state. They are typically interested in social interaction with their parents and peers, and while peculiar behavior can be seen, it is not an overwhelming characteristic.

The third, autism spectrum disorder, is characterized by delays in 3 cardinal areas of development: social interaction, communication/play, and stereotyped patterns of behavior. These children will often have marked speech delay and/or delays in global cognition. They will often have areas of strength, such as amazing puzzling skills, visual memory, or nonverbal problem solving. They have impairments in imitation, gesturing, and empathy and will often have marked obsessive and compulsive traits. The impairment in socialization carries the most weight when diagnosing a child with autism spectrum disorder, and the impairment should be above and beyond what the developmental age of the child would predict.

The early identification of developmental disorders has been a priority of pediatricians for many years. The balance of conservative management in those who show minor delays and the need for prompt recognition and further evaluation in those who have marked delays has been difficult to perfect. It is well established that the specificity/sensitivity of parental concerns of abnormal developmental trajectory is approximately 75% to 83% in detecting global delays in development in the child. Unfortunately the absence of parental concerns carries a modest 46% specificity of normal development. Parent report screening tools include the Ages & Stages Questionnaires–3 (ASQ-3), Parents' Evaluation of Developmental Status (PEDS), and Child Development Review–Parent Questionnaire (CDR-PQ) for general developmental concerns and the Ages & Stages Questionnaires–Social Emotional (ASQ-SE) and Modified Checklist for Autism in Toddlers (M-CHAT) for social and emotional concerns. Observational tools are for the health care provider to fill out and include BRIGANCE and the Denver Developmental Screening Test-II (DDST-II). The DDST-II has been found to have poor sensitivity and specificity and to identify only 30% of children with language impairments and 50% of children with intellectual disabilities. It is therefore not the first choice for developmental screening in recent years. If a child is found to have abnormal developmental trajectory on a general developmental screening tool, one should complete a more detailed screen for possible autistic features (see above). Due to the limitations of any one screening tool or parental questionnaire in finding all children who have delays in motor, speech, or social development, the combination of "listening to" parental concerns while independently "looking for" signs of delays is a vital combination for every physician and health care worker participating in the well care of infants and toddlers.

Every child with abnormal developmental screening should be evaluated by a physician with significant experience in early childhood development and referred for audiologic evaluation and lead screen. Further testing such as neuroimaging (magnetic resonance imaging/computed tomography), electroencephalogram, and genetic and/or metabolic testing should be considered but is not required for every child with mild/moderate delays.

A multidisciplinary approach is the preferred modality when assessing a child with developmental delays or possible autism. The most comprehensive evaluation would consist of a medical assessment, psychologic evaluation, physical and occupational therapy evaluations, an evaluation by a speech and language pathologist, and a parental interview with a social worker. Independent information of adaptive skills and behavioral difficulties should be obtained from daycare/school setting. Testing included in such an evaluation would include the following:

- Cognitive testing to evaluate verbal, nonverbal, and spatial reasoning skills. In school-aged children these tests also include assessments of working memory and processing speed. Such tests are standardized and include the Bayley Scales of Infant Development (BSID), Wechsler Preschool and Primary Scale of Intelligence (WPPSI), Wechsler Intelligence Score for Children (WISC), Differential Ability Scale (DAS), Stanford-Binet Intelligence Scale (SB5), Kaufman Assessment Battery for Children (K-ABC), and others.

- Speech and language evaluation to evaluate receptive and expressive language abilities.

- Adaptive behavior assessment to determine how the child responds to daily demands. Standardized tools include the Vineland Adaptive Behavior Scale (VABS) and the Adaptive Behavior Assessment System (ABAS).

- Autism evaluation tools include a parental interview to review the child's developmental trajectory from an autistic point of view. This tool, the Autism Diagnostic Interview (ADI-R), is a labor-intensive 2- to 3-hour interview although abbreviated questionnaires such as the Social Communication Questionnaire (SCQ) can be used in certain cases. The Childhood Autism Rating Scale (CARS) is a behavior rating scale that is extremely helpful in diagnosing autistic spectrum disorders. The gold standard for evaluation of autistic features in a child is the Autism Diagnostic Observation Schedule (ADOS), which is a direct observational tool where the child interacts with a skilled tester and the quality of social interaction/play and verbal and nonverbal communication is evaluated for autistic features. Autistic behavior checklists and Asperger symptom questionnaires also serve a purpose in screening those children in need of a full autism evaluation.

- Behavior checklists are valuable when assessing inattentiveness, hyperactivity, or disruptive behavior. These checklists include the Conners' Child Behavior Checklist (CBCL), the Vanderbilt, and other similar screening and diagnostic tools for parents and teachers.

- Motor developmental assessments include evaluations of gross and fine motor skills.

Children with developmental delays should be referred for early intervention services and these services should be tailored around the child's needs and social status. Most children will reach their highest developmental potential if they receive appropriate services and understanding at home and in school. Setting goals that are out of reach for the child or punishing them for lapses in behavior or academics will not lead to improvement, but celebrating every accomplishment will.

SECTION XII

UNUSUAL EPISODIC MOMENTS

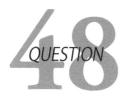

HOW ARE MOVEMENT DISORDERS CLASSIFIED AND WHY IS THAT IMPORTANT?

Jessica A. Panzer, MD, PhD

There are many causes of pediatric movement disorders, and they must be properly classified in order to guide appropriate evaluation and treatment. Some movement disorders are relatively benign (ie, a stereotypy in an otherwise healthy child), whereas some almost always reflect a pathologic process (ie, chorea). Movement disorders involve impaired performance of voluntary movements, abnormal postures, abnormal involuntary movements, or normal-appearing movements performed unintentionally.[1] Although they affect movement, spasticity, hypotonia, and weakness are generally **not** classified as movement disorders.[1]

Movement disorders are broadly divided into 2 groups: hypokinetic and hyperkinetic. Hypokinetic movement disorders involve too little movement, such as the bradykinesia seen in Parkinson's disease. These rarely occur in children and will not be considered further here. Hyperkinetic movement disorders involve unwanted or excess movements and are more common in children. They are caused by dysfunction of the motor pathways involved in the planning or coordination of movement, including the cerebral cortex, basal ganglia, brainstem, and cerebellum.[2] They vary markedly in terms of treatment, diagnostic evaluation, and prognosis—some of these disorders are quite benign, some are chronic and treatable, whereas others are neurodegenerative and ultimately fatal, and still others may be progressive but amenable to intervention.

Often, 2 or more types of abnormal movements (such as chorea and athetosis) exist in the same child. In addition, movement disorders may mimic each other or may mimic seizures. To make these distinctions, it is important to ask a series of questions when seeing a patient with abnormal movements, including the following[1]:

- Do the movements change over time?
- Can the movements be suppressed?
- Do the movements stop during sleep?

Licht DJ, Ryan NR, eds. *Curbside Consultation in Pediatric Neurology: 49 Clinical Questions* (pp 259-263). © 2016 Taylor & Francis Group.

- Is there anything that makes the movements better or worse?
- Are the movements present at rest or triggered by action?
- Is there a premonitory sensation or urge?
- Is the neurological examination otherwise normal?

Tics

Tics are "repeated, individually recognizable, intermittent movements or movement fragments that are almost always briefly suppressible and are usually associated with awareness of an urge to perform the movement."[2] Tics are further classified as motor or phonic, and as simple or complex.[1] Children typically have one or more repeated, distinct tics. Over months, a child's tic repertoire will change; individual tics will wax and wane. New tics may develop, and old tics may fade away. Stress, excitement, and fatigue can increase tics, and active engagement in a task may decrease them. Tics are typically suggestible and briefly voluntarily suppressible. Children may describe an urge or premonitory sensation that is relieved by performing the tic; this feeling increases if the tic is not performed.

Tics are very common and, almost always, are **not** a symptom of a serious neurological problem. Very rarely, tics are a sign of basal ganglia disease,[2] but there likely would be other concerning findings. In a child who has tics, a normal neurological examination, and an unconcerning history, no further testing is needed, although screening for commonly associated psychiatric comorbidities, such anxiety, inattention, or obsessive-compulsive disorder, should be conducted. Tics can mimic partial seizures, dystonia, myoclonus, or chorea—all of which would need further evaluation. The presence of suppressibility, a premonitory urge, lack of interference with ongoing tasks, and a clear beginning and end of each movement would point toward a diagnosis of tics. In addition, choreiform tics are more stereotyped than the random movement fragments of chorea.[2]

Stereotypies

Stereotypies are "repetitive, simple movements that can be voluntarily suppressed."[2] Most often these are rhythmic, bilateral movements of the upper body, such as hand flapping. In contrast to tics, stereotypies are more constant over time. A child will typically have a single movement type rather than an evolving repertoire of movements. Similar to tics, stereotypies can be increased by stress or fatigue, but they also tend to occur more often when a child is engrossed in an exciting activity. Although stereotypies may be suppressible, children do not describe a premonitory urge. The presence of suppressibility helps to distinguish stereotypies from other rhythmic movements such as tremor or myoclonus.

Although children with developmental disorders have an increased incidence of stereotypies, they also occur commonly in normally developing children—a fact that may need emphasis to avoid undue parental anxiety. Such children may be at increased risk, however, for the future development of tics, obsessive-compulsive behaviors, and attention deficit hyperactivity disorder.[3] Stereotypies tend to start a bit younger than tics, typically in toddlerhood or the preschool years. In a healthy child with a stereotypy who has a normal neurological examination, no further testing or treatment is needed.

Ataxia

Ataxia is "the inability to generate a normal or expected voluntary movement trajectory not caused by weakness or involuntary muscle activity."[2] It is discussed in Question 30.

Dystonia

Of the hyperkinetic movement disorders, among the most common to require further evaluation is dystonia. Dystonia is defined as "involuntary sustained or intermittent muscle contractions" that "cause twisting and repetitive movements, abnormal postures, or both."[2] These postures can replace or be superimposed on voluntary movements, and are often triggered by voluntary movements. The duration of dystonic postures can range from just a few seconds to hours or even be fixed, resulting in permanent contractures. Brief episodes of dystonia can cause a jerky tremor. Within each patient, there may be a characteristic posture or repertoire of overlapping postures. "Overflow," the regional spread of dystonia associated with voluntary muscle activation, is often seen. For example, an attempt to move the hands may result in dystonic posturing of the neck.[2] The absence of dystonia during sleep can help distinguish fixed dystonia from a joint contracture. Dystonia can sometimes be relieved by a "geste antagoniste" (sensory trick) such as lightly touching the chin to relieve torticollis.[1,4]

Primary dystonia is caused by a number of genetic mutations. Secondary dystonia is most often caused by injury to the putamen and globus pallidus. Other central nervous system regions can be involved, however, ranging from the corticospinal tract (including in the spinal cord), thalamus, cerebellum, and sensory cortex.[2] Hypoxic-ischemic injury to these regions, resulting in dyskinetic cerebral palsy, is a very common cause of pediatric dystonia. Secondary dystonia can also be caused by encephalitis, autoimmune disorders, structural lesions, strokes, metabolic disorders, and neurodegenerative diseases.[2] As these other etiologies have specific treatments, interventions, or prognostic implications, in the absence of a clear hypoxic-ischemic event, further evaluation is warranted.

Chorea

Chorea is "an ongoing random-appearing sequence of one or more discrete involuntary movements or movement fragments."[2] Individual movements can overlap and flow from one body part to another and can lead to the appearance of fidgeting. Children may try to incorporate chorea into purposeful movement (parakinesia).[2] On examination, there is motor impersistence. Findings include inability to sustain tongue protrusion and fluctuation in grip strength ("milkmaid's grip").[1,5] Chorea at the shoulder or hip, resulting in larger-amplitude flinging movements, is termed *ballismus*, and may be caused by lesions to the subthalamic nuclei.[2] Rapid, jerky chorea can be difficult to distinguish from myoclonus.[1] Chorea is more rapid, more continuous, and less stereotyped than dystonia. It is also less likely to be triggered by voluntary movements. Chorea is less sinuous and flowing than athetosis. Chorea is neither suppressible nor stereotyped, which distinguishes it from tics.[2]

Chorea can result from dysfunction of the cerebral cortex, basal ganglia, or thalamus. Encephalitis, autoimmune disorders, and toxic-metabolic encephalopathies (such as hyperthyroidism) can also cause chorea.[2] In children, the most common cause is Sydenham's chorea, associated with streptococcal disease and rheumatic fever.[5] Chorea may also have a genetic or neurodegenerative etiology. Given the important treatment and prognostic implications, it is very important to distinguish chorea from other abnormal movements, such as a choreiform tic.

Athetosis

Athetosis is "a slow, continuous, involuntary writhing movement that prevents maintenance of a stable posture."[2] It can be present at rest or with voluntary movement and is often more prominent distally. It is slower than chorea, and there are not discrete movement fragments. Unlike dystonia, there are not sustained postures. Athetosis most often occurs in combination with either chorea (choreoathetosis) or dystonia, and may be considered part of the spectrum between the 2 rather than a distinct entity.[1] It is most often seen in association with dyskinetic cerebral palsy or kernicterus.[2]

Myoclonus

Myoclonus is "a sequence of repeated, often nonrhythmic, brief shock-like jerks due to sudden involuntary contraction or relaxation of one or more muscles."[2] It can be focal, multifocal, or generalized. Sudden muscle contraction causes positive myoclonus, while sudden muscle relaxation causes negative myoclonus. Either type is followed by a slower return to the original position.[2] Myoclonus is also classified by its presence with action, sustained posture, or rest. Myoclonus and myoclonic seizures are not synonymous; generalized myoclonic seizures typically have an associated electroencephalogram correlate and originate in the cortex.[6] Repeated rhythmic myoclonus results in "myoclonic tremor," which is distinguished from true tremor by the presence of a fast and slow phase.[2] This distinction is important, as many causes of pediatric tremor are relatively benign whereas myoclonus is often more ominous.

Myoclonus can be associated with reversible metabolic derangements, such as the asterixis (negative myoclonus) seen in hepatic failure.[1] Benign causes of myoclonus include sleep myoclonus and benign neonatal myoclonus; myoclonic jerks are also seen in juvenile myoclonic epilepsy.[6] Otherwise, myoclonus is generally a concerning finding, often reflecting cortical gray matter dysfunction from metabolic disorders, anoxia, encephalitis, and neurodegenerative diseases.[2,6]

Tremor

Tremor is "a rhythmic back-and-forth or oscillating involuntary movement about a joint axis."[2] Tremor velocity is symmetric in both directions, in contrast to the fast and slow phases seen in rhythmic myoclonus. It is further classified as rest, postural, or action tremor. Intention tremor and dysmetria are distinct from action tremor. Associated with cerebellar dysfunction, these are defined by increased tremor amplitude with approach to a target. Dystonia can sometimes cause tremulous movements, but, compared to true tremor, these are more irregular and jerky.[2]

There are several relatively benign causes of childhood tremor, including enhanced physiologic tremor, shuddering spells, and essential tremor (typically with a family history). Some children with fine motor delays have an action tremor, especially with fatigue.[1] Psychogenic tremor is frequently seen, especially in teenagers. Hyperthyroidism and other metabolic derangements can cause tremor and should be ruled out. Pediatric head tremors such as spasmus nutans and bobble-head doll syndrome warrant central nervous system imaging.[7] Serious etiologies of tremor include Wilson's disease, other neurometabolic/degenerative diseases, brain tumors, and other focal brain lesions. A tremor that is disabling, present at rest, asymmetric, or associated with other abnormal neurologic findings should raise concern for a more serious underlying disorder and trigger appropriate investigations.

Acknowledgments

This work supported by National Institutes of Health grants T32DA022605 and K12NS049453.

References

1. Singer HS, Mink JW, Gilbert DL, Jankovic J. Classification of movement disorders. In: *Movement Disorders in Childhood*. Philadelphia, PA: Saunders/Elsevier; 2010:16-19.
2. Sanger TD, Chen D, Fehlings DL, et al. Definition and classification of hyperkinetic movements in childhood. *Mov Disord*. 2010;25(11):1538-1549.
3. Muthugovindan D, Singer H. Motor stereotypy disorders. *Curr Opin Neurol*. 2009;22(2):131-136.
4. LeDoux MS. Dystonia: phenomenology. *Parkinsonism Relat Disord*. 2012;18(Suppl 1):S162-S164.
5. Cardoso F. Sydenham's chorea. *Handb Clin Neurol*. 2011;100:221-229.
6. Lozsadi D. Myoclonus: a pragmatic approach. *Pract Neurol*. 2012;12(4):215-224.
7. Keller S, Dure LS. Tremor in childhood. *Semin Pediatr Neurol*. 2009;16(2):60-70.

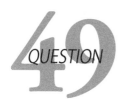

How Do I Diagnose Tics and How Do I Treat Them? When Is It Considered Tourette Syndrome?

Donna J. Stephenson, MD

Tics are abnormal, repetitive movements or sounds that are under only limited voluntary control. Tics are commonly classified as either motor (able to be seen but not heard) or vocal (producing an audible sound). Both types of tics are caused by sudden muscle contractions and share a similar pathophysiology. The most common presenting tic of childhood is probably eye blinking. Other simple motor tics include eye movements, mouth opening, facial grimacing, and neck jerking. More complex motor tics include slow and sustained (dystonic) movements such as brief torticollis, shoulder shrugs/rolls, and blepharospasm (forced eye closure). Simple vocal tics include sniffing, coughing, clearing the throat, and humming. More complex vocal tics include echolalia (repeating others' words), palilalia (repeating one's own words), and abnormal breathing patterns. Fortunately the most obtrusive tics such as coprolalia (obscene words) and copropraxia (obscene gestures) are not common, especially in childhood.

Tics are differentiated from other movement disorders by several features. In verbal children, a description of a premonitory urge to tic can be elicited and is very specific to tics. This can be perceived as a tightness in a muscle group, itch of the eyes, or funny feeling in the back of the throat. Once the tic is performed the urge is at least temporarily satisfied. Contrary to popular notion, tics can occur during sleep but are not as obvious as when awake. Tics are under some voluntary control, although it takes much concentration to suppress them. The onset can be abrupt or gradual. Tics are often more pronounced during times of stress, boredom, or fatigue. They are frequently reported to increase during sports and screen time activities. Tics wax and wane over days and weeks. It is common for one tic to subside and another, different tic take its place. Multiple tics can occur concurrently. It is most common for initial tics to be simple ones. Tics gain complexity as time goes on.

Tics usually begin between ages 4 and 6 years. Between ages 8 and 12 years, tics are usually at maximum intensity. In most teenagers tics begin to subside, and by age 18 50% are tic free. Tics

Licht DJ, Ryan NR, eds. *Curbside Consultation in Pediatric Neurology: 49 Clinical Questions* (pp 265-268).

can recur during adulthood, especially during times of stress. Boys are more likely than girls to develop tics. Conservative estimates of tic prevalence in childhood range from 5% to 10%; there have been some population studies suggesting the real prevalence is up to 25% but that most children with tics are not brought to medical attention. There is often a family history of tics or Tourette syndrome, but it may be forgotten if the family member's tics were transient and long ago. Genetic influence is probably multifactorial as no single gene has been implicated across several studies.

Most commonly, there is no underlying neurologic or systemic reason identified for the development of tics. Tics are seen frequently in conjunction with many types of developmental disorders. Maternal pregnancy and birth history should document prematurity, fetal distress, and neonatal neurologic syndromes that may lead to a static encephalopathy. A history of developmental delays or atypicalities should be solicited. Medications and recent medication changes may trigger tics in a susceptible individual. A review of systems should include screening for liver disease, birthmarks suggestive of a neurocutaneous disorder, seizures, and neurologic regression, which may indicate a more systemic disorder.

The physical and neurologic exam is usually normal in children with tics. The general physical exam should focus on growth and development as well as a thorough skin exam for neurocutaneous stigmata. The neurologic exam should focus on muscle tone, dexterity, and reflexes as well as tests of sequencing and motor movements to elicit soft neurologic signs and possible frontal lobe dysfunction. If the exam is normal and history is consistent with tics, then no further testing is indicated. An abnormal exam may warrant referral to a neurologist, magnetic resonance imaging, or other testing as indicated for metabolic or systemic disease.

There are significant comorbid neuropsychiatric conditions in 50% to 90% of children with tics. These include attention deficit hyperactivity disorder (ADHD), obsessive-compulsive disorder (OCD), anxiety, depression, learning disability, and developmental coordination disorder. It remains unclear whether autism is a comorbidity or a cause of tics but the 2 disorders do appear commonly together. These disorders all need to be screened for in the history as they may result in more functional problems than the tics themselves. Treatment of the comorbidities can result in increases or decreases to tics in an unpredictable way.

Tourette syndrome is a specific form of a childhood-onset tic disorder. Criteria for Tourette syndrome include the presence of multiple motor and at least one vocal tic occurring over the course of at least 1 year with no tic-free intervals longer than 3 months. A diagnosis of Tourette syndrome does not change the likelihood of remission, which remains at 50% by age 18. Tourette syndrome is treated only as needed in the same way tics are treated (see Treatment of Tics).

In the last 20 years an entity known as Pediatric Autoimmune Neuropsychiatric Disorders Associated with Streptococcus (PANDAS) has been proposed as a specific disorder commonly presenting with childhood-onset tics. The description is of otherwise healthy children who very abruptly develop a constellation of tics, obsessive-compulsive behaviors, and anxieties in the setting of a resolved or active strep infection. Evidence for the existence of this disorder is lacking, as multiple investigators have failed to elucidate a specific antibody response or biomarker that is specific and sensitive for this disorder. Proposed treatments have included moderate and long-term use of prophylactic antibiotics as well as more conventional psychotropic medications targeting specific neurologic symptoms. Immunotherapy has been used in suspected cases but is not currently recommended. At present most neurologists do not feel that PANDAS is a diagnosis apart from more common childhood disorders and do not prescribe antibiotics for treatment of tic disorders.

Treatment of Tics

Not all tics require treatment. Often demystifying tics and Tourette syndrome to caregivers and patients is the most important job of the physician. Reassuring parents of the benign and developmental nature of the disorder can be all that is required. It is wise to adopt a "wait and see" approach if the tic is not causing a problem for the child. I do counsel patients not to help the child "break" the habit with reminders or prompts to stop the tic. Bringing attention to the tic, which is often not even noticed by the child, may in fact lead to an increase in tics as a child's anxiety level rises.

Tics do require medical treatment if they are problematic for the child. Tics can cause physical symptoms such as neck pain, headache, and eye irritation. Tics can result in low self-esteem, anxiety, and bullying. Treatment of a comorbid condition such as ADHD may be very effective and necessary but can be associated with exacerbation of an underlying tic disorder. In that instance, the tics may require treatment as an acceptable side effect of the medication for the comorbid condition.

Pharmacologic treatment of tics consists of neuroleptics and other medications. Currently only 2 medications are Food and Drug Administration (FDA) approved for the treatment of tics: haloperidol and pimozide. Improvement of tics with neuroleptic medication has been recognized since the 1960s. There are rare but serious side effects associated with neuroleptic use. Atypical neuroleptics such as pimozide or risperidone are preferred as they have a lower chance of precipitating extrapyramidal movement disorders. In general, non-FDA-approved, milder medications are usually used as first-line therapies. A list of medications is listed in Table 49-1, from most to least commonly used.

The alpha adrenergic agonists clonidine and guanfacine have been studied and are used as first-line medications. They are effective in reducing tic frequency and severity with a good safety profile. Guanfacine is often preferred as it may cause less sedation. Rarer side effects include mood changes and dizziness. Clonidine is often beneficial for sleep-onset trouble, often seen in children with comorbid anxiety and ADHD. As it can cause more sleepiness than guanfacine, clonidine is often used only at night or with half doses during the daytime hours.

Topiramate is being used with increasing frequency despite lack of controlled studies demonstrating efficacy in children. The dose range is lower than used in epilepsy so the medication is usually well tolerated. Side effects include parasthesias, fatigue, cognitive dullness, kidney stones, and decreased appetite.

Other medications include low-dose baclofen and clonazepam. Onabotulinum toxin can be used for extreme and troubling motor or vocal tics.

Medications should be used for as long as necessary. After a period of weeks or months of tic quiescence, an attempt should be made to gradually taper and discontinue the medication.

A specific form of cognitive behavioral therapy, habit reversal therapy, has been studied and is effective at tic reduction in older kids and teens with specific troubling tics. Currently providers trained in the methodology of habit reversal are rare in community settings.

Comorbid conditions such as ADHD and OCD should be addressed with medication and behavioral strategies as indicated. Although the FDA has warned against treatment of ADHD with stimulant medication in the setting of tic disorder or Tourette syndrome, more recent studies have refuted the notion that stimulants consistently worsen or cause tics. Atomoxetine, a selective noradrenergic reuptake inhibitor, is also appropriate for the treatment of ADHD and does usually not affect tic symptoms. Selective serotonin reuptake inhibitor medications are indicated for the treatment both of OCD and anxiety.

Table 49-1
Commonly Used Medications for Tic Suppression

Medication	Usual Dose Range	Common Side Effects
Guanfacine	0.5 to 2 mg daily	Sedation, constipation, dizziness
Clonidine	0.05 to 0.2 mg daily	Sedation, constipation, bad dreams
Topiramate	15 to 100 mg daily	Parasthesias, fatigue, mental fogginess, renal stones
Baclofen	2.5 to 20 mg daily	Fatigue, weakness
Clonazepam	0.5 to 2 mg daily	Fatigue, irritability, dependence
Risperidone	0.25 to 2 mg daily	Weight gain, dystonia, metabolic syndrome
Pimozide	0.5 to 5 mg daily	Weight gain, QT interval prolongation
Haloperidol	0.5 to 5 mg daily	Weight gain, extrapyramidal movements

Suggested Readings

Jankovic J, Kurlan R. Tourette syndrome: evolving concepts. *Mov Disord.* 2011;26(6):1149-1156.

McNaught K, Mink JW. Advances in understanding and treatment of Tourette syndrome. *Nat Rev Neurol.* 2011;7(12):667-676.

Piacentini J, Woods DW, Scahill L, et al. Behavior therapy for children with Tourette disorder: a randomized controlled trial. *JAMA.* 2010;303(19):1929-1937.

FINANCIAL DISCLOSURES

Dr. Laura A. Adang has no financial or proprietary interest in the materials presented herein.

Dr. Robert A. Avery has no financial or proprietary interest in the materials presented herein.

Dr. Ernest Barbosa has not disclosed any relevant financial relationships.

Dr. David Bearden has no financial or proprietary interest in the materials presented herein.

Dr. Timothy J. Bernard has no financial or proprietary interest in the materials presented herein.

Dr. Lauren A. Beslow has no financial or proprietary interest in the materials presented herein.

Dr. Diana X. Bharucha-Goebel has not disclosed any relevant financial relationships.

Dr. Lori L. Billinghurst has no financial or proprietary interest in the materials presented herein.

Dr. John M. Binder has no financial or proprietary interest in the materials presented herein.

Dr. Jason Coryell has no financial or proprietary interest in the materials presented herein.

Dr. Louis T. Dang has no financial or proprietary interest in the materials presented herein.

Dr. Mai T. Dang has no financial or proprietary interest in the materials presented herein.

Dr. Renée A. Shellhaas has no financial or proprietary interest in the materials presented herein.

Dr. Maximillian H. Shmidheiser has no financial or proprietary interest in the materials presented herein.

Dr. Laufey Yr Sigurdardottir has not disclosed any relevant financial relationships.

Dr. Karen L. Skjei has no financial or proprietary interest in the materials presented herein.

Dr. Douglas Smith has no financial or proprietary interest in the materials presented herein.

Dr. Donna J. Stephenson has no financial or proprietary interest in the materials presented herein.

Dr. Christina Szperka has received grant support from Pfizer, which makes topiramate, one of the preventive medications mentioned in Question 19, and was a site PI for the NIH-funded Childhood & Adolescent Migraine Prevention Study comparing the effect of amitriptyline, topiramate, and placebo in migraine prevention.

Dr. Katherine S. Taub has no financial or proprietary interest in the materials presented herein.

Dr. J. Michael Taylor has no financial or proprietary interest in the materials presented herein.

Dr. Christian Turner has no financial or proprietary interest in the materials presented herein.

Dr. Amy T. Waldman has no financial or proprietary interest in the materials presented herein.

Dr. Ryan P. Williams has no financial or proprietary interest in the materials presented herein.

Dr. Courtney J. Wusthoff has no financial or proprietary interest in the materials presented herein.

Dr. Michele L. Yang is currently a PI on a study sponsored by Pfizer and a co-I on a study sponsored by Sarepta. She was previously a PI on a study sponsored by Santhera.

Dr. Sabrina W. Yum has no financial or proprietary interest in the materials presented herein.

INDEX

Printed in the United States
by Baker & Taylor Publisher Services